Introduction So here we are with the third or fourth attempt at completing this project of the Reality Weight Loss Program. To be honest I am not sure why every other attempt at completing this has failed. I have begun to wonder if it was because I had not truly committed to my own weight loss. What ever is the reason for this, I am at it again and 1hopefully I will complete everything this time.

I want to first take this introduction to explain my reasoning for doing this the way I have. I am forty-four years old at the time of writing this and I can honestly say that I am in a place that I have not been in a long time. Although, my weight is not where it needs to be I am the lowest that I have been in almost fifteen years. I am weighing in at 268 lbs, and I have dropped almost five sizes in the last few months.

In saying this I will admit that I am still battling diabetes and struggling with a high cholesterol reading. This is where I am at this time in my life. Yet, I give God glory that the battle that I had fought with my blood pressure has been won.

Emotionally I am presently struggling with some hard issues in my personal life but the move to Florida has been helpful. I have chosen to make this a place where I am rebuilding my life; physically, emotionally, and spiritually. In doing this I have chosen to start this project again and establish a local Bible study/ prayer meeting for those who are struggling with these issues.

So here I am working on this project and I want to say thank you to specific people who have played a part in this projects completion. To my Lord Jesus

Christ who has set me free from the bondage that held me for most of my life. To Him and Him alone be the glory and honor.

To my family, thank you for your encouragement and support. I know that my moods have been on a rollercoaster ride as I have struggled through this weight loss and you have loved me through it all.

To my son Nathan, who traveled with me to Florida. You have been my strength and support in the hardest times of my life. You came and worked out with me and helped me stay on track, even though you occasionally helped me cheat. I love you son.

To my friend, and helper, and companion, you know who you are and I say thank you for being there when I needed you. You kept me focused on the true prize.

To my brother, friend, pastor, Curt you will always be my best friend. I know that I can be a pain, but you still loved me and spoke the truth even when I didn't listen. Thanks.

And to you my reader and compatriot in this battle. Thank you for being here and reading this book. Thank you for fighting the fight and being a voice to all those who battle with obesity.

R.

My Story:

I am the fourth child born to James and Imogene Simmons. In my life I have always been a big kid and have struggled obesity. Much of my life was spent trying weight loss program and after program and failing. The hardest part of all these programs was that they were not based on the real world. These programs, as good as the were, never dealt with the real issue in an overweight persons life. They never dealt with the whole person.

As I was growing up, I held within myself this image of my worth. It was frail and weak. It was based on all the ridicule that I heard from the kids at school, the teachers, even my family members. I held that image and it daily beat me to death.

There were moments of victory that I can remember. There were times when I actually took great strides in winning this battle with my weight. But I still never confronted the real beast that held me in bondage.

It was many years later in my life that I stood and looked at a full length mirror and saw myself. "Randy," I said, "Your not overweight, your not chubby, or husky, or large, you are fat and either loose the weight or die." This moment of revelation was the first step in winning this battle. But don't get me wrong it wasn't complete.

I spent the next few months working on loosing weight. I started the Slim Fast program and was also using Dexatrim to help. (A combination that I would not recommend.) And by late 1988, I had lost a large amount of weight. I was hitting the gym in Melrose Park, II, real hard and had lost probably around

35lbs. But the problem was that I was doing things the wrong way and harming my body.

I would eat extremely small meals for breakfast and lunch, then hit the gym for two hours. I would come home and have only a salad, then do push-ups and sit-ups before going to bed. This lasted for almost six months but the first chance I got I fell back into old habits.

The real problem was that I never dealt with the core reason for my weight. I was treating only one part of my true self. It wasn't until six years ago that I came to realization of the truth in this. I had been off my diet for many months and had put a large amount of weight back on.

I had hit the heaviest that I had ever been in my life (432lbs). I was diagnosed with diabetes, and high blood pressure. I had even had a close call with an inflamed gall bladder. As I lay on the emergency room bed, the doctor came in and told me a hard fact. I had been in the emergency with the same symptoms three times and they had not been able to find any problem. This particular time they had used a different examination tool and had found the problem. As the doctor looked at me he said that it was because of my extreme obesity that they had not been able to find the inflamed gall bladder.

Even with all this information I still continued with my eating habits and lack of exercise. But God has to, some times, hit us with a bat to make us wake up, and that is exactly what He did.

As I was driving to work one day I noticed things were very blurry in front of me. I felt that this was something that I should take seriously and went to the local Urgent Care. They did a series of tests and in a few moments the doctor came in to talk with me. She didn't soften the truth.

"Mr. Simmons loose weight or die!!!, Your sugar was so high that the meter could not read it, your blood pressure is high enough that we were surprised that you had not had a stroke. The fact is that if you continue with what you are doing, you will be in here in a couple months either in a coma or suffering a stroke."

That doctor saved my life. The truth was painful but it woke me up. I didn't want to miss out on the life of my children or my grand-children. I knew exactly what I needed to do. I set my course and despite all the obstacles and times that I fell, I have kept the course.

I tell you these things because I want you first to understand that I have been there and I am still battling. This is a day to day fight that is more than just pushing the plate away. It incorporates the full person that you are.

I had to come to a realization that my victory needed to involve every part of my life. It required a complete change in all of my life. It was a mental choice to pick up that chocolate bar or that cookie. In the same manner it would take a mental choice to say "NO".

There were also spiritual issues that had become part of my thought process that I had to deal with. The image that I had allowed to take root in my thoughts had to be changed. I needed to realize that I was created in the image of Christ. Knowing this that everything that God created He said was good, meant that I was good.

Does this allow me to abuse my body with bad food or lazy behavior? No, it instead pushes me to correct my failures and bring my body back to the place that God had intended it to be.

I find myself in a time of great struggle. My wife has filed for divorce, I am in a new place and around strangers. All of these things have begun to push me toward the triggers that have been the sources of my obesity.

You may ask why I am being so transparent. Well, dear reader, I want you to see the ground work that I believe is the Reality Weight Loss. These truths are based around the fact that we are a three part creation. This means that we are physical, emotional, and spiritual creatures.

So how does this apply to weight loss and health? Well, let me lay out some simple guide lines that we will use as we go through this program. In it I will show you just how each part fits together to accomplish weight loss and victory in your life.

You are a physical being:

·You require proper nutrition

·You require proper activity

·You require proper medical input

You are an emotional being:

·You require emotional input

·You require mental stimulation

·You require emotional support

You are a spiritual being:

·You require a spiritual relationship

·You require spiritual nutrition

·You require spiritual awakening

With each of these parts I want to impress on you, dear reader, that it requires of you a complete lifestyle change for it to work.

I do want to prepare all of my readers to understand that my personal faith will be incorporated within my teaching. This is because I believe that obesity is much more than just a physical issue. I believe that obesity is mainly a spiritual issue. Therefore, to see ourselves completely changed, and health to be restored we need to deal with these spiritual issues.

Now as you continue to read through this program and, hopefully begin to put it into practice, I trust that you will begin to see a change in your life.

Always remember, dear reader, that weight loss is 90% mental and only 10% physical. This means that the greatest hindrance to your victory is you. Make the choice to overcome your obesity, no matter the cost, and you will win.

YOU ARE A PHYSICAL BEING

We understand that our physical body has been created to accomplish certain things. To maintain this goal our body is in need of three main ingredients.

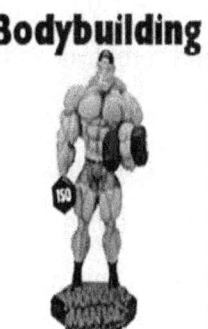

Bodybuilding

·**We require proper nutrition:**

This means that to maintain our daily activity and mental capacity we need to have a certain amount of vitamins and minerals taken in on a daily basis. The problem is that the average American doesn't take in the correct amount of vitamins and minerals. Those of us that battle obesity have this intake of vitamins and minerals so badly thrown out of balance that we often struggle with other physical issues.

Proper nutrition for each person is often different. Many of us have an imbalance of minerals or vitamins resulting in high cholesterol or diabetes. We may struggle with poor bone strength or ulcers. Many of us have high blood pressure. Each of these can be determined by a physician.

A good diet is the most important part of this. Many of us have tried to loose weight through starvation diets or fad diets. This is another example of the improper nutrition. The problem with many of the diet plans out there is that it causes your body to be thrown out of balance. They ask you to cut your calorie input to bare minimum or eliminate some other nutritional element that can cause you to fall back into starvation mode. This is a point in our physical make up that the body begins to store fat instead of burn fat. It may even result in our body burning muscle tissue.

A proper diet plan is actually a balanced calorie intake, with a low sugar and carbohydrate intake. You should actually have eight small meals in the day and stop eating at least two hours before going to bed. There needs to be a high intake of liquids, preferably clear liquids. With this it is required that you have at least twelve glasses of water (8 oz.) each day. It is also suggested that you have a daily vitamin with each meal.

I have included in this book a diet plan that lays out some suggestions to help you with your daily menu. In this I give some ideas for each meal but I am not laying down any rules. These are only suggestions to help. I have also included some recipe ideas that have given me some change in the bland menus that usually accompany diet plans.

·We require proper activity:

Exercise is the most important element in a diet plan. This is because the body cannot burn off fat tissue without an increase in metabolism. This increase will not occur without the body having some activity to bring the heart rate and body temperature up.

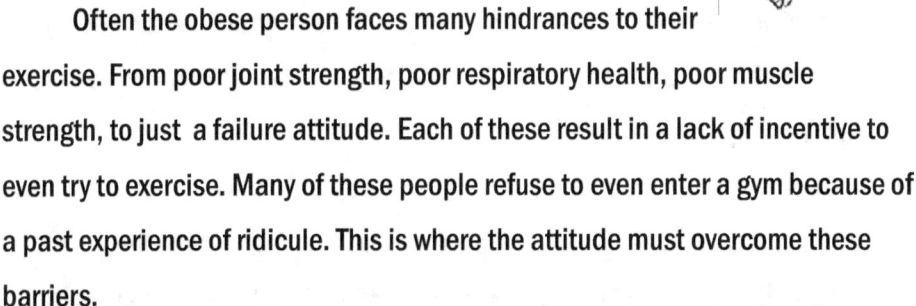

Often the obese person faces many hindrances to their exercise. From poor joint strength, poor respiratory health, poor muscle strength, to just a failure attitude. Each of these result in a lack of incentive to even try to exercise. Many of these people refuse to even enter a gym because of a past experience of ridicule. This is where the attitude must overcome these barriers.

Any form of exercise will begin the process needed. I have even given suggestions for those who do not or can not use a gym to simply begin with standing up a few times, then do "push-aways" from the wall. These will begin building in the body the needed changes in metabolism. The result will be a slow increase in respiratory health, joint strength, and muscle endurance. Each of these will help to accomplish the needed change.

An important fact for you dear reader is that I ask you to begin by consulting your physician before you start any type of exercise program or weight loss program. Each of us have physical limitations and you need to keep your doctor informed about any thing that you are doing that may result in a radical change in you body.

I have laid out an exercise plan that is a good starting point for you to work with. I suggest that you begin each morning with some simple knee bends, push-ups, and sit-ups. Keep your goal simple and don't strain yourself. For those of you who cannot do a full sit-up, refer to the diagram in the Exercise chapter for alternative ideas. Each of the beginning exercise ideas has an alternative movement.

I have also shown you a set of goals and with each goal is an advancement in the see ourselves completely changed, and health to be restored we need to deal with these spiritual issues.

Now as you continue to read through this program, and hopefully, begin to put it into practice, I trust that you will begin to see a change in your life.

Always remember, dear reader, that weight loss is 90% mental and only 10% physical. This means that the greatest hindrance to your victory is you. Make the choice to overcome your obesity, no matter the cost, and you will win.

·We require medical input:

It is my opinion that a person who is obese is a fool if he fails to get medical care. A simple check up can be the one element that can save his life. The doctor can discover anything from diabetes to high blood pressure or may even find that you have a thyroid imbalance. These may give you vital information to assist in finding that freedom from your obesity.

The other element of the medical input may also be a psychological input. Many of us not only struggle with obesity, but depression or low self-esteem. These issues can be sources to finding answers to our problems.

Medical input can help with your ability to exercise without getting injured. Knowledge of joint issues, damaged tendons, or poor muscle tone may prevent you from causing a more serious injury.

Knowledge is power in your weight loss. And in this battle you need all the knowledge that you can obtain to win. The help of your family doctor can be crucial in your battle.

Get your doctor involved in your weight loss. From the point of your first weigh-in to your monthly check-up. Have the doctor monitor your progress so that he can use it to encourage others.

I had an endocrinologist (diabetes doctor) suggest that I talk to her patients because I had gotten control of my diabetes. She wanted me to tell them that it could be done with just a proper diet and good exercise.

I want to make it clear that you are a physical being that requires proper activity, nutrition, and medical input to be in balance. These elements will bring your body back to the place that God intended it to be. When we are in balance we will find more than just weight loss, we will find peace.

YOU ARE AN EMOTIONAL BEING

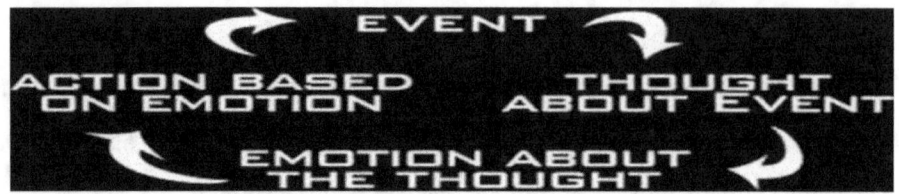

The human being is more than just tendons, muscle and bone. We are emotional beings. We require mental stimulation and nurturing. We require person to person contact and acknowledgment for our accomplishments. Each of these elements can often be found missing in an obese persons life.

These factors may be a cause or just the result of their destructive lifestyle. So to face these truths is to overcome a missing part in your life.

·We require emotional input:

One of the biggest struggles that I had in my journey was proper emotional input. This missing element held me back from victory over my weight for many years.

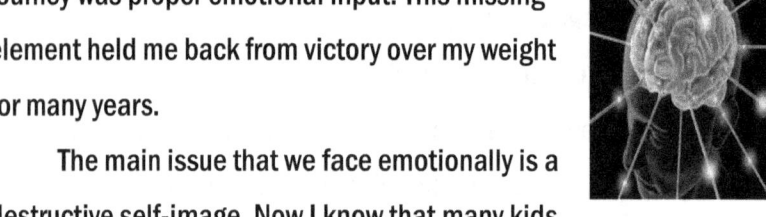

The main issue that we face emotionally is a destructive self-image. Now I know that many kids have been ridiculed for most of their school life for their weight. I was one of them. The issue is that this self-image carries over into our adult life and we constantly find ourselves replaying the ridicule in our heads.

This becomes a trigger to our eating habits. It pushes us to failure in our diet and often in our daily life. We need to turn this around and tell ourselves that those people are going to be eating their words when they see how you look after you reach your true body weight. Take a photo of where you are now and prepare to take another one in three months.

Believing that you have worth is a daily change of attitude for many of us. What I suggest is that you take a moment every morning and stand at the mirror. While you are there I want you to say this simple set of words.

"I have been created in the image of God. Because of that I am created to accomplish great things. I am a person of value and worth. I am loved by the Creator of the Universe. I know that if I were the only person on the face of this earth, Christ would have died for me. I know that He has promised to set me free from my mountain and therefore I know that He sees worth in me. God doesn't make junk, therefore I am not junk. I am good, cause God said I was good."

Now as foolish as you may feel the first time, continue to do this. As you do, you will find that your whole attitude will change. You may find that you will need to do this more than once a day. That is okay. You are going through a process of changing your perspective of yourself.

One part of this rebuilding yourself emotionally is going to be dealing with some of the memories that will begin coming to the surface. Our memories have a powerful effect on how we view ourselves. They can unconsciously manipulate our clothing choices, our friendships, our employment choices, even our eating habits.

I would make a suggestion that you may want to seek a psychological counselor to help you deal with some of these memories. I have done this and have found myself experiencing great healing. The counselor that you choose can help you take each memory and deal with it as you are able. They can also help you find freedom from its control of your life.

Another method of dealing with these memories is to keep a daily journal of your personal feelings as you go through this diet program. Remember that you are a three part being. You are going to be needing to confront some painful things in your life if you truly want to experience freedom.

As you begin working on this daily journal, keep track of your weigh-ins and your daily exercise plan. Also keep notes on your personal feelings as you begin your day and end your day.

Has the day been a good day? Did you stay on your diet or did you cheat and how did it make you feel? Did you remember someone that may have hurt you with words? Do you need to forgive that person? Do you need to talk to that person?

Each of these questions will need to eventually be answered. Now, I am not suggesting that you call up every kid that ever teased you in school. I am instead suggesting that you take a time to write their name on a piece of paper and look at it. Take the time to remember what they did and how it hurt you. Now I want you to take that paper and place it in a bowl. Light the paper on fire and watch it burn. As it burns I want you to say these words...

"Lord, (their name) really hurt me. Those words were painful and they cut me deep. But I know that my words have hurt You, many times. And yet, even though I hurt You and deserved Your wrath, You forgave me. So God, I give (their

name) to You. I forgive them, as You have forgiven me. I release my anger. I ask that You will forgive me for holding this anger. I ask that You will bless (their name) with all that they need in their life. Bless their family. Bless their work. Bless their finances. I thank You Lord for my freedom, AMEN."

Will this be easy? Absolutely not. This may be the hardest thing that I have asked of you. Yet, I will tell you that you will feel a freedom like never before.

You may feel the need to call this person and just ask them to forgive you. If it has been a long time, just let them go. Yet, some of us have had this verbal abuse even in our adult life. So do whatever the Lord directs you to do.

Another part of this process is dealing with our self-destructive behavior. We are causing our bodies harm as we eat. This self-destructive life is something that we need to confront with honesty. The main problem is that it will find a way to show itself no-matter how hard we try to avoid it. So admit this to yourself and talk to your counselor with honesty.

I had to admit that I was trying to kill myself. Every time that I engulfed two Big Macs, fries, and a coke, I was trying to kill myself. I knew what it was doing to my body. I knew that I was heading to the grave. Yet I continued. Why? Because I did not see any worth in my life.

Friend, we cannot try to cling to ignorance as an excuse. We are not ignorant of what grease, and fat, and cholesterol does to the human body. We know that it will eventually clog arteries, and kill us. We are suicidal and that is the truth.

A person who is obese is killing themselves every time they ignore their doctor and refuse to go on a diet. Just admit it, dear reader, and stop. You want to live. You want to be free. You want to be healthy. That is why you picked up this book.

Triggers tell us volumes about our reasons. Identify what your triggers are emotionally. Many of us deal with depression. This is a powerful trigger that will push us into our bad eating habits.

Depression has been my own trigger for many years. I find myself heading that direction when I am struggling financially or presently when I deal with my ex-wife. In those times I find a way to pull myself into the arms of my Lord. I spend time praying or reading my Bible.

Another method of overcoming this trigger that I use is going to the gym. I find that I experience a release in my body that brings me emotionally up out of my depression and I can begin to refocus my thoughts toward positive things. But for each of us it is different.

TRIGGERS:

There are three main topics that are triggers for the average person. They show themselves in different ways but usually are rooted in...

BOREDOM: Most obese people have a problem with motivation. This is often referred to as stagnation. Many of them battle with bad joints, poor muscle strength, poor respiratory and cardiovascular health. These battles provide them an excuse (although a poor one) to remain sitting on a couch or in bed. Overcoming this is a key point in finding their freedom from obesity.

DEPRESSION: Depression can kill a person faster than a bullet. I truly believe this to be fact. So many people find themselves buried in a deep debilitating depression. It can keep them locked within their homes, their minds, their own world. I believe that this is one of the biggest issues that many obese people hide from their family and friends.

STRESS: Stress is a killer of many Americans. We battle stress over finances, marital issues, our children, war, crime, even international issues. But how many of these things can we truly change in our selves? Can we honestly have any effect over the international issues of war, or our social problems? Yet, stress will push many of us to overeat.

The real problem is that we need to have some kind of emotional control over our lives and we feel that we have lost this control. So the only thing that we know we can control is our eating. Yet, we find our own eating habits have gotten out of control, and the triggers sound.

Emotionally we are in desperate need of help if we are going to find the freedom that we need.

·We require mental stimulation:

Being that we are emotional beings, we are often lacking in mental stimulation. But what could I be meaning by mental stimulation? Simply put this means sitting down and reading a book.

So often we will find ourselves sitting in front of the television with our mind in a haze. We are earnestly seeking some kind of thought provoking program and finding only brainless blather. Yet we remain glued on the sofa, our eyes locked on the show, as our brain turns to mush. Suddenly, we crave food and the cycle begins.

Why do we allow this to happen? Because we are hungry for input, but it is not for body food. Instead, our body is hungry for emotional and mental food. We are needing to feed our brains with something other than the latest American Idol.

The mind needs to be stimulated for it to grow and mature. Kids today are suffering from the highest rate of obesity than ever before. The reason for this is that the average child spends more time in front of the television than they do reading a book.

Children feel that they can substitute their need for mental stimulation with time on the internet and still they are obese. This is because the internet does not stimulate their imagination. I found myself in that trap at an early age. I found myself lost in TV shows and cartoons. Yet, I remember the times that I didn't sit in front of a television and went outside to explore lost worlds and build wild inventions.

Where had that time gone? It was lost to shows like "The Six Million Dollar Man", and "The A-Team". I didn't need to imagine those strange new worlds when the television did it all for me. And our children have fallen into the same trap. The internet has taken the need for imagination out of the hands of our children and replaced it with virtual reality. Our adults are the product of an imagine-less world. That is why so many of us are suffering from obesity, boredom, and poor health. We never get out of our chairs or go for walks. We never pick up a book and read it. Instead, we would rather sit in front of the TV and let it do all the work for us.

So, enough talking from my soap-box, and let me suggest some solutions to this problem. I want to suggest that you set a goal to read at least two books each month. Begin with this goal and try to increase it every other month. I would suggest that in that goal you would include reading through the Bible in a year. There are many Bible study plans out there that help you accomplish this. Go to your local book store and you will find them.

I have attempted this many times and failed, but I did start. So I have laid out some ideas to help you. Check out the chapter "Bible Study" and you will find my suggestions. I have also listed some resources to help you with going through the Bible. Along with this I would suggest that you choose a devotional. This is a good start to your morning. It helps deal with that emotional baggage. It will help you keep your mind in focus and away from distractions. What ever you choose to read through, just do it.

Another form of emotional stimulation is some kind of hobby. Even exploring the art galleries. This will open up your mind to new ideas and new experiences. We have remained hidden for too long and that is why we battle depression. Bring out the old guitar or the drawing pad. Let your creative side explode into new areas that it has never gone. Put your thoughts into a book that tells your story. Each of these things will begin feeds that part of you that has been starving.

·We require emotional support:

I have mentioned this previously but I do want to go back over the issue of a counselor one more time. We are emotional creatures. This means that we have baggage, both good and bad. This baggage has a way of controlling our response to moments in our lives.

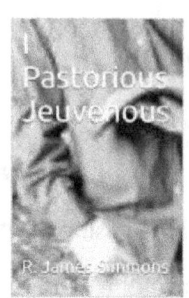

I have co-written a book called, "I Pastorious Jeuvenous." This book is a biography of pastors son that went through many things. In this book I talk about this persons life after, sexual abuse, pornography addiction and many other things. These events shaped the way that the man dealt with stress and struggle that he faced later in his life.

We need to understand that the events of our past effect our future. Therefore if those events were painful, they can have a way of pushing us toward self-abuse instead of self-worth. The words of ridicule from a family member can destroy a child and result in a self-destructive lifestyle.

Because of all this, it is helpful to find someone that you can open up with and talk through these memories. There are many Christian counselors out there that have a big heart and desire to see you set free.

Another source for you emotional support is your pastor. Take the time to sit down with your pastor and tell them about what you are doing. Explain what I have shared in this book, even let them read through it, so that they will understand how you want to deal with all of your stuff.

You may want to search for a twelve step group that is Christ based. Get with a group of people that are going through the same thing that you are dealing with. Use them to help you with emotional support. And as you open up you will find freedom.

<u>YOU ARE AN SPIRITUAL BEING</u>

The hardest truth for me to accept is that obesity is sin. Therefore this meant that I had to accept that my eating habits were sin. *"But I don't go out and choose to gorge myself,"* you may be saying. I am not going to apologize in saying that , yes you do.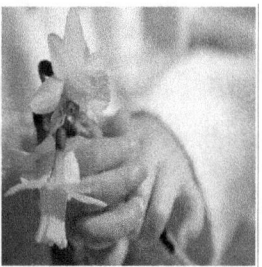

Every time that you sit down to eat, no matter if it is good food or bad, you make a choice. No one forces you to eat those ten "fig nutins". No one shoved that entire chicken down your throat. You made a rational choice to eat that food. Therefore, you made a choice to go against the plan of God.

But, dear reader, do not be discouraged. Know that we serve a merciful God that understands our struggles. He knows our frailties and is compassionate toward us.

What I needed to understand was that I had allowed the enemy to take up a stronghold in my life, in the area of my eating. I also had to understand that this stronghold was not just in my eating, this was the result of the original stronghold. The true stronghold was deep in my own self-image.

In allowing the enemy to control my self-image, I had also given him control over what I did with my own body. This lead to many other struggles that have resulted in my own self– abuse issues.

The first thing that I needed to do was recognize that I had to put God back in His rightful place in my life. He was Lord of my life and I had to give Him complete control of every area that was me. This wasn't easy and it has been a daily battle but each day that I allow Him reign, I have victory.

So, dear reader, let me take you through this return to Lordship, so that you can find the same freedom.

·We require a spiritual relationship:

The simple question is, how can God be Lord of your life if He has never even had a place in your life? Therefore the logical first step is to recognize your need for Him to set your free.

The greatest day in my life was when I understood my need for salvation. That was the day that Christ took up residence in my life. I found a friend like no other. He didn't laugh at me when I failed, nor did he accuse me when I deserved it. Instead He offered and showed me unconditional love.

My father had demonstrated this love to me as I had sat in rebellion and demanded to go out on my own. Despite the fact that I deserved his hatred, my father knelt before me and began to pray. That was love. The same love was shown to me, as Christ hung on a cross that I deserved. He could have rightfully called the angelic host of heaven to destroy all of mankind, yet He prayed to His Father that He would forgive us.

If you desire to experience true freedom in your life, call out to God for His love to be shown to you. As you do, confess that you are a sinner. **"But I haven't** killed anyone, or stolen, or any of those real bad things, I'm good," you may be saying. But have you ever told a lie? Then you deserve death.

"For the wages of sin is death, " This is the law of God. If you have sinned (broken the law of God) then you deserve death. We all deserved death. "but the gift of God is eternal life in[b] Christ Jesus our Lord.(Romans 6:23 (New International Version)

This is God's mercy. "But God shows and clearly proves His [own] love for us by the fact that while we were still sinners, Christ (the Messiah, the Anointed One) died for us." (Romans 5:8 Amplified Bible)

Each of these scriptures tells us that we need a savior. How can you turn away from such love? This is the most rational thing for us to accept. Life or death which will it be for you?

If you are willing to take that first big step to freedom and accept the gift of God, the scripture also tells us this truth... "For God so greatly loved and dearly prized the world that He [even] gave up His only begotten ([a]unique) Son, so that whoever believes in (trusts in, clings to, relies on) Him shall not perish (come to destruction, be lost) but have eternal (everlasting) life" (.John 3:16 (Amplified Bible)

The average obese person is facing a life with only ridicule to look forward to. Who would willing go into that life without a true friend? Christ can be your true friend. And in being that true friend, He is willing and ready and able to set you free from the bondage that has held you for all your life. That bondage that is your eating habits.

He can and will release you from those memories. He will heal you from those emotional hurts. He will heal you from those physical issues that have held you bound to failure. He desires total freedom for you and for me.

Pray this prayer with me and lets take this first step to our spiritual freedom...

"Lord God, I understand and confess that I am a sinner. I see that I am without You and without You I see that I can not have life. I now accept the gift of Your Son Jesus Christ and the sacrifice that He gave on the cross. I release control of my life, my eating habits, my thought life, and my self image. I accept that You have created me to experience the joy that You have for me. I ask that You take Your rightful place in my life as Lord and Savior. I rejoice that I am now free from sin, and have a promise of eternal life with You, AMEN."

If you have prayed this prayer I want you to understand that you have not begun a religious experience but a relationship. You have stepped into the presence of the Creator and He has adopted you into His family. Therefore you are a new creation and all that old life is now gone and you have a brand new life.

This is the Reality of a spiritual relationship. You can now experience joy and freedom in this new life. You don't have to be bound up by the past. You can let it go and give it over to your heavenly Father.

But what about those of you who have already had this life change? What has gone wrong with your spiritual relationship?

Let me tell you something that I had to admit to myself. I am not perfect. Shocking as that was to my overgrown ego, it was the truth. I am not perfect, but Christ in me is. He has given me a new life and I had just left it sitting on the kitchen table. Oh, don't get me wrong, I preached about this new life and I sang about it. I even wrote a few songs about this new life, but I had yet to experience the reality of it in my daily walk.

I needed to experience a spiritual awakening. And, dear Christian brother or sister, this is what you need to experience. You need an awakening. You need to stop beating yourself up about all those things that you have failed at and messed up. Pick up the scripture. Fall to your knees. And cry out to the Lord God. No excuses, no formula, no pretense, no King James prayer. Just cry out.

Do you want freedom? Then cry out to God and say, *"Lord God, set me free! I am tired of trying to do this on my own! I can't do this anymore! Help me! I give up! I need Your help!."*

"There is therefore now no condemnation for those who are in Christ Jesus…" Is this true? Of course it is. You are a new creation. Why are you still under condemnation?

Guilt is part of religion. You have been given a relationship. Jesus Christ came to be your Lord. He has called you His child. He has placed within each of us His Kingdom. He has given us the Holy Spirit who constantly does intercession for us. He has promise you that He will return for you. All these things should change your perspective. This is a relationship.

My lesson for you in this section is to take your journal and write the following words in bold ink. Don't be shy about it. Tell the whole world. *"I am a child of the Most High God. I have been adopted into His heavenly family. I stand on the promise that He has made to come back for me and bring me into His heavenly Kingdom, so that where He is I will be forever. I have been made above and not beneath. I am created to praise Him and praise Him I will, with all that is in me I will praise Him. I have been made the head and not the tail. I have been promised that whatever I ask of Him, He will do that His Father may be glorified in me. All these things are mine in Christ Jesus. Therefore I am made complete in Him and I am now no longer under the condemnation of sin, I am a new creation my old life is passed away and behold all things have been made new."*

Declare these things as you write them and begin to declare them on a daily basis as you start your day, as you declare your daily affirmation. I promise you that you will see a change in your day.

·We require spiritual nutrition:

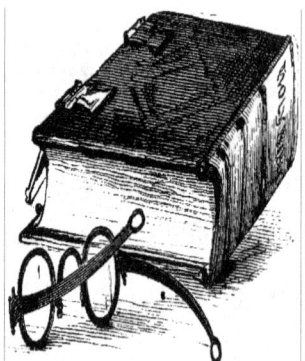

What are you feeding your spirit man on a daily basis? Sadly, most Christians have minimal or even no devotional life. They attempt to make it through their daily walk with only the previous Sunday School lesson, or sermon to support them. They rarely have a prayer life except for the occasional "fox-hole" prayer and then they wonder why they have no power.

I faced this reality as I have been going through one of the hardest times of my life. My battle with obesity was nothing compared to the recent battle for my marriage. I was left homeless and unemployed.

In one week, my home was gone, my family abandoned me, and I found myself in a new state, a new home, and among strangers. I faced all this with nothing to call a prayer life or devotional support. I was trying to overcome a spiritual desert and found myself suffering spiritual malnutrition.

In the same way that your body cannot survive without food. Your spiritual life cannot survive the daily battle without being fed daily.

This truth is one that I had heard so many times as I grew up in church. So often, those dear spiritual grand-parents would try and get me to take home a devotional guide and I would just smile. "They think that I need that? Oh, good grief, don't they realize that those things are for the young Christians. I am a powerful man of God. Can't they see that?"

The reality is that I was arrogant and trying to live off of the food I got on Sunday. Yet when the real battle came at me I had nothing to hold on to. I would strain and stretch for those few small morsels to try and gain some strength. And occasionally they would get me through the battle but I would end up bruised and torn and weak.

If you want to avoid those times and want to find true balance in your daily walk, then I suggest that you prepare to start a daily Bible study. In doing this you may want to ask friends to join you. Gather up some additional material to help you work your way through the scripture.

There are many resources to help you. I have included a daily devotional in this book to help you get started. It will give you, also, a resource guide to find other devotional material.

The goal here is to change your patterns. Now, there are not many devotional resources specifically designed for those struggling with obesity. I hope to write out a full devotional guide and make it available from my publisher. But until that day comes, use the chapter that I wrote to get things started.

Another part of your spiritual nutrition is finding a good church. Now there are those who believe that they can make it through their life without the input of any spiritual food, even Sunday. But I am here to tell you that they are fooling themselves. The scripture commands that we not "forsake the gathering of yourselves together." Those times of worship and fellowship are crucial to the success of this program. Because it is here that you will find the support to make it through the hardest times.

You are battling a spiritual war, dear reader. This is not just a physical change. If you truly want this to be a permanent change in your life then you need to understand that there is more to this than just a diet.

When you come to church and begin to worship, you can experience spiritual refreshing and restoration. You will also have the opportunity to allow people to pray with you. Know that prayer is also a crucial part of this program.

Communication with the "manufacturer" is important for a mechanic to have any chance of restoring a car. Therefore if you want to see true freedom from this monster, than you need to have time to pray. Ask God to show you the many areas that you will need to change. Many of these specific areas will be completely unique to you. He knows your life. He knows your thoughts. He can show you things that only you will understand.

Another element of this spiritual nutrition is to gather people around you who can daily lift you up in prayer. The power of prayer partners is immeasurable. Those friends who will keep you in prayer as you work through each of your areas will be key elements to your success.

Keep these people on a prayer list. Notify them when you have victories and failures. Tell them the times that you feel the most temptation to fail. Let them know when you will be going to your doctor, or counselor. These things may be areas that they will feel a need to pray.

·Give them the tools that they can use to help you through this time in your life.

·We require a spiritual awakening:

I have hinted at this but I will talk about it 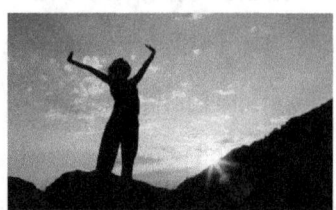 again. The fact is that we all need a spiritual awakening. The United States is no longer anywhere close to being a Christian nation. This is seen in our movies and in our daily lives. The media has become a place of sex, sex, and more sex. We sell even the most innocent products with sex.

The worst part of all this debauchery is that our children have become the victims of our sin. The scripture tells us that "the sins of the fathers will be visited to the third and fourth generation." We can see this in the lifestyle of the average school child.

But how is this related in the dietary lifestyle of the modern day American? Simple, we have become a nation obsessed with itself. Our arrogance can be seen in the magazines, television, and movies.

The children of our nation have become grossly overweight or suffer from malnutrition. We have kids killing themselves to stay thin. Our teen boys are popping as many diet pills as the average suburban housewife did in the fifties. They workout in the gym to the point that they have no social life. Or they gorge themselves on fast food, beer, and candy till they suffer heart attacks at the age of twenty.

And where is the church in all this? Sadly we are the worse of the bunch. The average church attendee is at least fifty pounds overweight. The pastors are so out of shape that many of the health insurance companies will not cover them for fear of early death. Many of them suffer from high blood pressure, diabetes, and heart problems.

The average teen in church has no activities and will only attend church if they are having free food. They are often extremely over weight and have few social contacts. They often suffer from low self-esteem and have considered suicide.

The sad state of our churches in American screams at us that we need an awakening. But what do I mean by awakening? I would describe it as God slapping us awake to see the state that we are in. We need to wake up.

How does this happen in the individual? How do we awaken to our own spiritual condition?

Well, the first step is to pick up a book like this and say, I want to change. This tells me that you are tired of the "same old stuff" and see the need for change. If this is your heart cry then you are heading in the right direction.

The next step is to say that you want God to have His way in your life, no matter what it may cost you. This may require that you give up some things that you have held on to for all your life.

When you make that choice to allow God free reign in your life you are returning His rule over everything. A king in the medieval times had the freedom to do whatever he may have chose to do with his kingdom. If he chose to sell off a piece of land he could do that because he owned everything. But what does this mean for you and I?

This means that if God chooses to send you to talk to that mean neighbor, than He can do that. If He tells you that you need to stop drinking Cokes, then He can do that. Why? Because He is Lord of your life, and this means that you are not living your life, but Christ is living in and through you.

Do you hunger and thirst after His righteousness? Do you desire to see Him glorified in your life? Are you willing to surrender your will to His will?

If you can say yes and yes again, then you are ready to experience a spiritual awakening in your life.

Let's take this first step and pray a simple prayer....

"Lord God, I come to you with all those things that I have wanted in my life. I recognize that these are my wants. I am ready to lay all of these things down and let You have them. I lay each part of my life before Your throne, Lord. I lay down my appetite. I surrender my diet . My physical self belongs to You. My emotional wants and needs are no longer mine. Lord, I give up my friends, my family, my past relationships, my present relationships. They are all Yours now Lord. I lay down my spiritual struggles now Lord. All of my questions. All of my sin and failures. They are not mine anymore. I am empty before You God. Completely and totally empty. Now God, I ask that You come in and awaken me. Give me Your eyes and Your heart. Let me see myself and others as You see them. Stir up within me a fire, like never before. Place within my heart a hunger and

thirst for You. Give me Your passion for the lost and hurting. Give me Your

passion for my health; emotionally, physically, and spiritually. And Lord I will

give You and You alone all the glory."

If you have prayed this prayer than don't leave your new fire at the kitchen table. Take this awakening out to your church or those friends that are praying for you. They need to know that the awakening has begun in your heart and it is time to take it to the whole body of Christ. Your new found freedom needs to inspire the hearts of the body of Christ. You can be a catalyst to start a revival for this generation. Let the Word of God be alive in you so that you can spark the light in others.

<u>MYTHS</u>

In this chapter I want to dispel some of the myths that our society has perpetrated concerning the obese person. As I go through many of these myths I will hopefully provide you with information to prove the falsehood of these tales. These myths have caused many obese people to feel that they have no escape from their bondage. I hope that in this you will see that you can be free and find real health in your life. We understand that man has been obsessed with the human form for many years.

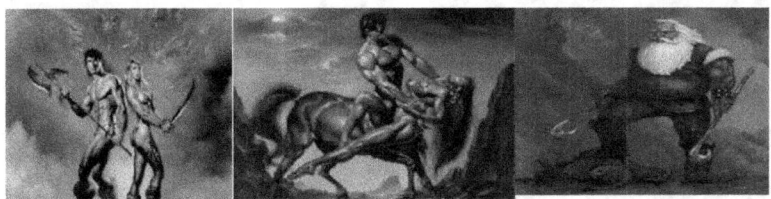

In our artwork and sculptures we see many obsession with the human form. In these pictures by Boris Valejo we can see how many people view the perfect form. Both Boris and his wife Julie Bell are famous for painting their images with extreme detail and using themselves as models. I chose these artists because I wanted to show how the image of a perfect form can differ when put against another interpretation.

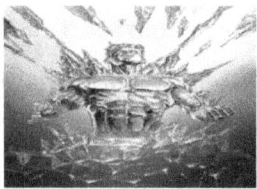 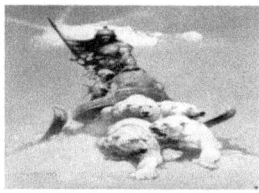 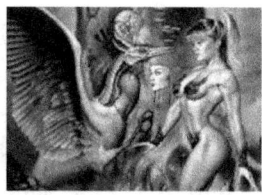

For example the Santa Clause is done by Frank Frazetta. His interpretation of the human form is quite different from Valejo and Bell. Frazetta tends to hide the form behind other things, whether clothing or animals. But in each of these pictures we can see how man views the form in specific ways. Still, we may ask ourselves, what is the true human form? What makes the correct form for me? Should I be buff and cut like one of these barbarians or trim and sleek like one of the ladies? What is the true human perfection for me?

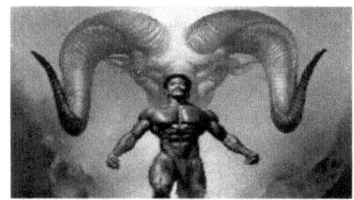 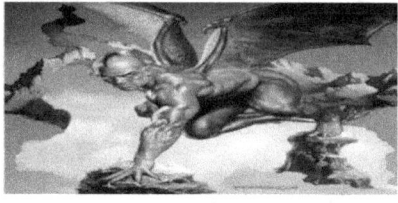

The myths of our society have pushed us into a self-indulgence social view of our bodies. We either have no concern for our appearance or we become so self absorbed that we are compulsive about our appearance.

In an article in Bodybuilding.com, the writer declares that we are fighting a new "battle of the bulge." In the article he says....

Amongst the adult population, figures are more dismal. According the CDCP (1999), 61% of U.S. adults are obese or overweight. In the United States, this pandemic shows indicators of record growth for the future. In other parts of the world, particularly in Asia, the problem of obesity is on the rise. In the Cook Islands 44% of women were obese in the 1960's. In the year 2000 this level rose to 57% (Easen, 2002). Despite the extensive knowledge available to our post-modern society, our problems are moving faster than we can catch them. An alarming percentage of the population is <u>obese</u> and out of shape; so much so that dieticians and doctors have borrowed the name of a World War II military campaign to describe their war on obesity: Battle of the Bulge." (© Bodybuilding.com, 305 Steelhead Way, Boise, ID 83704 USA - 1-877-991-3411)

The writer goes on to explain that the issue of obesity is not just a physical problem. It is a condition of cognition and emotion. This is to say that emotion is not a biological urge brought about by the action of neurons. Emotion is produced from a mental thought that causes a reactive condition.

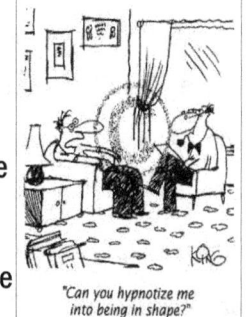
"Can you hypnotize me into being in shape?"

The emotion about a specific subject can control the actions of an obese person. This is why I mentioned about the need for emotional healing. But the writer of this article continues to provide a crucial look at the obesity situation in the United States.

"The amount of control one has over ones life is determinative of a person's level of self-esteem. Put another way, when one is in control of ones life, one feels well and secure. Because an obese persons low self-esteem stems from feelings of little or no control over life's "circumstances", people who are obese often experience feelings of helplessness, hopelessness and worthlessness. While this is not always the case, it is true more often than not. I have yet to hear of an obese person being overjoyed in the streets because of their condition and its resulting physical health complications. Cases of the obese being overjoyed about their condition are the exception rather than the rule.

The emotions that one has about being obese stem not from the condition, but from thoughts of lack of control over ones life, and the contrast resulting from physical comparison beside other people.

As mentioned, society places heavy emphasis on being thin and lean. Advertising and the media function as the consciousness of the nation; the supplement industries $5 Billion annual sales are a testament to the desire amongst the masses to be lean and fit. Traditionally, human beings have sought to have "ideal" figures. The ancient Greeks made statues of Hercules and other gods who were muscular and lean, and science has formulated mathematical tools like the BMI [Body Mass Index] to indicate an "acceptable" and "healthy" weight range for a person based on their height and body composition." (© Bodybuilding.com, 305 Steelhead Way, Boise, ID 83704 USA - 1-877-991-3411)

I would recommend that you read through some of these articles and check out their information yourself. I found them vitally helpful in my research for this book.

Another resource was the New Orleans Center for Eating Disorders. In their article I found a list of seven myths that they address. I would like to use these myths to go through this chapter. Now understand that there are many other misconceptions about obesity and obese people that society has created. These seven are just some myths that will help us get started.

Myths about Obesity

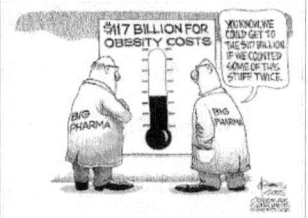

"**Myth 1: Body fat is unhealthy**: Actually, some body fat is essential and beneficial. For example, fat on the thighs and hips are reported to lower the risk of cardiovascular disease and type 2 diabetes, especially for women. A certain amount of body fat is necessary for normal body functioning. Too little can lead to infertility and osteoporosis."

This myth has propagated the faulty images that many of our teen girls have about themselves. The worse part of this misconception is that it can induce bulimia and anorexia. These compulsions have resulted an many young girls being hospitalized or dieing.

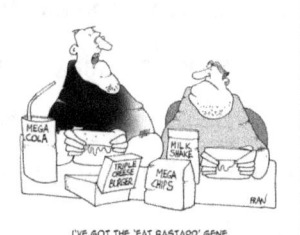

"**Myth 2:Obese people are at greater risk for cardiovascular disease**: Recent studies show that there is no connection between clogged arteries and obesity. In fact, fat on the body and fat in the bloodstream are different. Having more body fat does not contribute to increased fat in the arteries. Having excess caloric intake coupled with increased saturated fat intake can, however, increase arterial fat deposits."

Education can be the key to overcoming so many misconceived ideas about obesity. To understand your medical condition is to be armed for battle. Know your body. Know your medical problems so that you can battle them correctly.

"Myth 3:Weight loss improves health & lengthens life: Weight loss does not necessarily improve health or lengthen life. In fact, yo-yo dieters and those whose 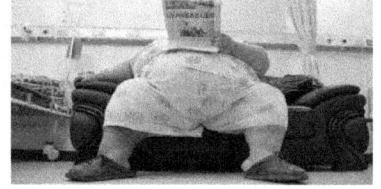 weight fluctuates throughout their adult lives are twice as likely to develop cardiovascular disease and type 2 diabetes than people who remain overweight."

It is necessary to include dieting and exercise to your daily activity but to maintain this lifestyle throughout the rest of your life. Remember that I told you at the beginning of this book that I was setting you for a complete change of life. This is exactly what I am preparing you for. Be sure to understand that this is not 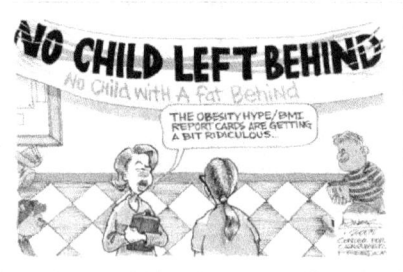 a cure all that will be a one time thing. You will need to maintain this change of life through out if you expect to avoid these potential problems.

"Myth 4:Obese people eat more than non-obese people: By 1979, 19 studies had already found that obese people eat the same or less than thin and normal weight people. Recent studies published in the American Journal of Clinical Nutrition and the Journal of Applied Behavioral Analysis

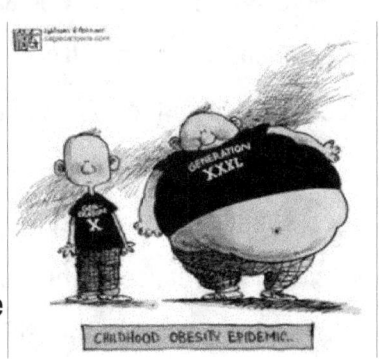

confirm these findings. Obesity is multi-determined, and eating is only one of the factors affecting one's weight. Genetics, endocrine function, activity level, lifestyle, medications and metabolism all play a role in determining a person's weight."

It is strange to think that for almost two years my intake of food was down to a bare minimum and yet I remained excessively overweight. The problem is that I had no activity to speak of and my body had stopped processing my calorie intake correctly. Many of us are confused because we feel that we are not eating as much as everyone else. Well the truth is that you very likely are not eating as much as someone else.

"Myth 5: Obese people are lazy and unfit: Many people who are classified as obese or overweight exercise regularly and are physically fit. These individuals have lower all-cause death rates than thin people who do not exercise and are unfit."

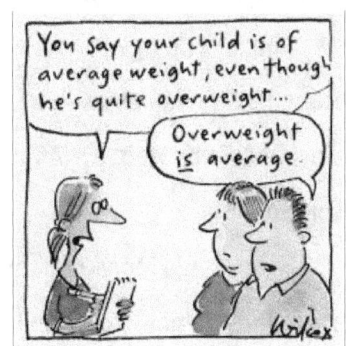

There are some people who are out there who are overweight that exercise on a regular basis and are still overweight. The average power lifter may be considered obese and yet works-out like a bodybuilder.

"Myth 6: Obese people are at greater risk for all diseases: Actually, overweight and obese people have lower risks for lung cancer (in both smokers and non-smokers) and osteoporosis than thin or average weight people."

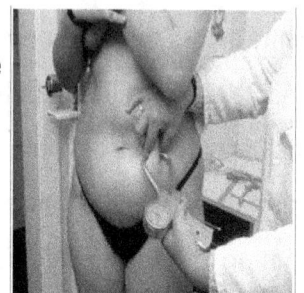

There are many people that assume that every potential disease is going to somehow be thrown upon people who are overweight. This is foolish. However, many obese people are susceptible to these diseases if they add to their problems by smoking or drinking. The individual that suffers from diabetes has a lower immunity level.

"Myth 7: Everyone gets fat with old age: The reason that weight can increase with age is because people are often less active and tend to lose muscle mass, which causes metabolism to slow."

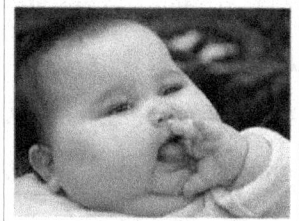

Obesity and age have no connection. Obesity is based on either metabolism, or inactivity. If, even the elderly, will keep their activity level up they will avoid gaining weight. (All content ©2004 New Orleans Center for Eating Disorders)

The average individual does not truly understand the life of an obese person. They do not know the depression, or the stress that we battle with on a daily basis. This feeds the mythology around obese people.

But one of the issues today is that it has become big business. Obesity and weight loss has become a multimillion dollar investment. You don't find many diet products that are inexpensive and this has resulted in a profit run mentality for the average weight loss corporation.

Friedrich Asen wrote an article entitled, "Myths About Obesity Like to Control You" In this article he expresses his frustration with the profit motivated weight loss program and how they seek only to take your money and not truly help the person.

"Weight loss and obesity are big business. Here are some factors that can make you rich if you happen to start a business related to weight management. Two thirds of America is overweight. Out of that, 50% are obese. 300.000 premature deaths are caused by obesity. Obesity is the fastest growing epidemic in the world. The world is hurling towards obesity at galactic speeds. Only 50 years back obesity was hardly heard of. Nearly 45% of the world population is obese or overweight in 2004.". © 2007 WebRing Inc

"This has far reaching consequences, of which these two seem to be of utmost importance.

1. If the motivation is business, the expert will not really be interested in healing the client, because that will harm his business.

2. If the motivation is business, he wants the client to stay dependent on him and his means (remedies, methods etc.)

The inevitable consequences of this are: The expert will favor a type of research that brings about medicines, drugs, devices and treatment methods, which will...

a. ...relieve the symptoms of the client by psychic and physical manipulation.

b. ...lead to a permanent dependency on the supply of this means. © 2007 WebRing Inc

It is my motivation in gathering this information for you, dear reader, to provide you with the tools to avoid these type of people. I hope that together we can both find the true healing that we both need.

Mr. Asen has provided crucial research into the motivation behind many of the weight loss charlatans that are taking advantage of obese individuals. He continues to share his heart in this article. It is clear that he has become equally frustrated with society and their view of obesity as I am.

"But you, dear friend, you have to wake up to your own intelligence and power. I shall give you a hint to the root of every problem: Wrong decisions on your part. Learn to correct them, and you'll start to get better immediately. Find a person, which you have trust in. Pray for guidance. You will be helped, whatever your problem is.

Do you really think that you can overcome obesity or any disease or problem by simply taking some pills or talking to a person, who is mainly interested in his own business?

Listen to this: "Current and past medical research has shown us that obesity isn't entirely due to unhealthy living; it is also influenced by our DNA. People who have had members of their family that have suffered from being overweight or obese will be at a high risk level of suffering the same problems and therefore need to take extra steps to help prevent that from happening."

I'll ask you just one question: Who makes up your DNA? Chance? So, let's fix it, the scientist thinks, lets do some genetic research and manipulate it.

I'll tell you, what your DNA is: It simply is the physical expression of your thinking, feeling and willing. And that you can change for the better, if you want. And if you need some support on the physical plane: There are hundreds and thousands of natural medicines, which will do a much better job than pharmaceutical poison.

"Delphine Eberle's work (Diabetes, Aug, 2004), with the sterol regulatory element binding protein transcription factor, found that the two isoforms are linked to the 'plasma leptin concentrations in American obese families.' His group hypothesized, '...genetic variations of the SREB-1 gene could be associated with obesity and obesity-related metabolic traits such as insulin resistance, type 2 diabetes, and dyslipidemia.'

Interestingly, SREB-1 gene polymorphisms were found among obese cohorts when compared to non-obese cohorts. This means they are on to something and possibly not far from marking the SREB-1 gene as a clear link to obesity (1)." See, "his group 'hypothesized' that something 'could be'". This is science. "Maybe, could be, perhaps..." All they want to say is that it is not you, who is in charge, it is the SREB-1 gene. It controls you, and now we will figure out to control it back.

This is simply nonsense. Are you a machine or a person endowed with free will? Decide for yourself. ObesityKiller.com. © 2007 WebRing Inc. "

Amidst all of Mr. Asan's rambling it is clear that he, in some way understands that obesity is more than just a physical issue. The truth, no matter how painful it may be, is that it is a spiritual issue. Obesity is sin. There may be some memories behind it; there may be even some physical issues involved, but it will always come back to, "I want my way."

The biggest myth out there is that it is not your fault. Remember that I told you that you had a choice. Well, you had a choice if you were to pick up that extra donut or cookie. No one forced you to eat those multiple donuts or candy bars. You made the choice to do this and therefore you are now in this condition and you can now choose if you want to loose weight.

I have said it before and I will say it again, "there is no secret pill or diet plan that will make you be thin and fit in twenty-four hours". It does not exist and if you read it in the newspaper or see it on TV it is a lie. There is no super diet plan that will make you loose weight overnight.

It is hard work and filled with many failures and trials. But if you will put your mind to it and set your mind in place, you can and will be free from this monster.

The reality is that you will have to change your whole life and start over.

The reality is that you will have to deal with some issues that have placed you on this destructive path.

The reality is that if you will make this choice and keep to it no matter what comes along, you will be remade into a new person, free from guilt and failure.

Will you be an Adonis? Or another Pamela Lee? Sorry, that isn't reality. But you will find the person that God had planned for you and you will see that He doesn't make junk.

DEFINITIONS

Okay I have bombarded you with so much information that your brain is probably heading into overload. Therefore I have decided to focus this next chapter on defining for you some of the terms that I have been using. Hopefully I will also provide you with additional information that will help you understand a little more about this creature we call obesity.

Our first definition is the topic of this book and that is obesity. What defines being obese? What is the usual characteristic of a person that is obese? And what are some of the results of being obese? Now I am going to gather much information to answer these questions. So I will have a section at the end of this chapter that will provide you with all of my sources. So be patient if you are keeping track.

Obesity (medical condition): Obesity refers to being more than 20% over your desirable weight. Unfortunately, it is all too common in the developed world where our modern lifestyle tends to make us eat more and move less. (Source: WD Writers)

Obesity: Excessive fat accumulation in the body.

Obesity: more than average fatness

Source: WordNet 2.1

Obesity: Is a Body Mass Index (BMI of 30 or above). BMI describes body weight relative to height and is strongly correlated to total body fat content in adults. The risk of death increases as the BMI reaches and surpasses 30.

(CDC98)

Source: <u>Diseases Database</u>

Obesity : excessively high accumulation of body fat or adipose tissue in relation to lean body mass; the amount of body fat (or adiposity) includes concern for both the distribution of fat throughout the body and the size of the adipose tissue deposits; individuals are usually at high clinical risk because of excess amount of body fat (BMI greater than 30).

Source: CRISP

Understanding Adult Obesity: NIDDK (Excerpt)

To most people, the term "obesity" means to be very overweight. Health professionals define "overweight" as an excess amount of body weight that includes muscle, bone, fat, and water. "Obesity" specifically refers to an excess amount of body fat. Some people, such as bodybuilders or other athletes with a lot of muscle, can be overweight without being obese. (Source: excerpt from <u>Understanding Adult Obesity: NIDDK</u>)

NIDDK _ Statistics Related to Overweight and Obesity: NIDDK (Excerpt)

Overweight refers to an excess of body weight compared to set standards. The excess weight may come from muscle, bone, fat, and/or body water. Obesity refers specifically having an abnormally high proportion of body fat. One can be overweight without being obese, as in the example of a bodybuilder or other athlete who has a lot of muscle. However, many people who are overweight are also obese. (Source: excerpt from <u>NIDDK _ Statistics Related to Overweight and Obesity: NIDDK</u>)

Obesity: Differential Diagnosis

Exogenous obesity (most common) –No demonstrable disease as the cause –Excessive weight gain from imbalance between caloric intake and energy expenditure –Linear growth is robust and frequently accelerated

Hormonal causes –Associated with poor linear growth –Hypercortisolism: Cushing syndrome is any type of glucocorticoid excess (endogenous or exogenous); Cushing disease describes pituitary ACTH overproduction –Hypothyroidism –Growth hormone deficiency

Insulinoma

Hypothalamic obesity –Tumors (e.g., craniopharyngiomas) –Following neurosurgery or irradiation –Head trauma –Infiltrative/inflammatory

Genetic syndromes –Prader-Willi syndrome –Laurence-Moon-Bardet-Biedl syndrome –Alström syndrome –Cohen syndrome –Down syndrome –Carpenter syndrome –Grebe syndrome –Beckwith-Wiedemann syndrome

Defects in metabolic/eating regulatory pathways is an area of intense investigation; multiple mutations are theoretically possible, but only a few have actually been discovered in humans –Congenital leptin deficiency (extremely rare) –Leptin resistance (more common than deficiency)

Drugs –Chronic glucocorticoids –Neuropsychotropic medications

Adiposogenital dystrophy syndrome

Obesity: Causes and incidence

Obesity results from excessive calorie intake and inadequate expenditure of energy. Theories to explain this condition include hypothalamic dysfunction of hunger and satiety centers, genetic predisposition, abnormal absorption of nutrients, and impaired action of GI and growth hormones and of hormonal regulators such as insulin.

An inverse relationship between socioeconomic status and the prevalence of obesity has been documented, especially in women. Obesity in parents increases the probability of obesity in children, from genetic or environmental factors, such as activity levels and learned patterns of eating.

Psychological factors, such as stress or emotional eating, may also contribute to obesity. Rates of obesity are climbing, and the percentage of children and adolescents who are obese has doubled in the last 20 years.

Causes: Obesity: Although some obesity is caused by **underlying disorders,** the main cause is probably lifestyle. The problem has two basic issues: too much food, too little activity. High calorie diets from processed foods and fats make it easy to add weight. Sedentary lifestyles without adequate exercise make it hard to take weight off. Evidence suggests that obesity has more than one cause: genetic, environmental, psychological and other factors may all play a part. (Source: Genes and Disease by the National Center for Biotechnology)

Article excerpts about the causes of Obesity: Understanding Adult Obesity: NIDDK (Excerpt)

In scientific terms, obesity occurs when a person consumes more calories than he or she burns. What causes this imbalance between calories in and calories out may differ from one person to another. Genetic, environmental, psychological, and other factors may all play a part.

Genetic factors

Obesity tends to run in families, suggesting a genetic cause. Yet families also share diet and lifestyle habits that may contribute to obesity. Separating these from genetic factors is often difficult. Even so, science shows that heredity is linked to obesity.

In one study, adults who were adopted as children were found to have weights closer to their biological parents than to their adoptive parents. In this case, the person's genetic makeup had more influence on the development of obesity than the environment in the adoptive family home.

Environmental factors

Genes do not destine people to a lifetime of obesity, however. Environment also strongly influences obesity. This includes lifestyle behaviors such as what a person eats and his or her level of physical activity. Americans tend to eat high-fat foods, and put taste and convenience ahead of nutrition. Also, most Americans do not get enough physical activity.

Although you cannot change your genetic makeup, you can change your eating habits and levels of activity. Try these techniques that have helped some people lose weight and keep it off:

Learn how to choose more nutritious meals that are lower in fat.

Learn to recognize and control environmental cues (like inviting smells) that make you want to eat when you're not hungry.

Become more physically active.

Keep records of your food intake and physical activity.

Psychological factors

Psychological factors may also influence eating habits. Many people eat in response to negative emotions such as boredom, sadness, or anger.

Most overweight people have no more psychological problems than people of average weight. Still, up to 10 percent of people who are mildly obese and try to lose weight on their own or through commercial weight loss programs have binge eating disorder. This disorder is even more common in people who are severely obese.

During a binge eating episode, people eat large amounts of food and feel that they cannot control how much they are eating. Those with the most severe binge eating problems are also likely to have symptoms of depression and low self-esteem. These people may have more difficulty losing weight and keeping it off than people without binge eating problems.

If you are upset by binge eating behavior and think you might have binge eating disorder, seek help from a health professional such as a psychiatrist, psychologist, or clinical social worker. (Source: excerpt from Understanding Adult Obesity: NIDDK)

Obesity: NWHIC (Excerpt)

The main causes of being overweight or obese are eating too much and/or not being active enough. If you eat more calories than your body burns up, the extra calories are stored as fat. Everyone has some stored fat. Too much fat results in being overweight or obese. Other factors that may affect your weight include your genes (obesity tends to run in families), your metabolism (how your body processes food), your racial/ethnic group, and your age. Sometimes an illness or medicine can contribute to weight gain. Researchers are studying the causes of obesity to learn more about how to prevent and reverse it. (Source: excerpt from Obesity: NWHIC)

Obesity is a condition of having excess body weight. When an adult is more than 100 pounds overweight, they are considered morbidly obese. In the U.S., 97 million adults are overweight or obese. Being overweight significantly increases the risk of death from hypertension, dyslipidemia, type 2 diabetes, stroke, osteoarthritis, coronary heart disease, gallbladder disease, sleep apnea and respiratory problems, and endometrial, breast, prostate and colon cancers. Obesity results in an approximate cost of $117 billion in the U.S.

Obesity has reached epic proportions. Rates of obesity have gone up from 12 to 20 percent of the population since 1991. This epidemic is not limited to adults: The percentage of young people who are overweight has more than doubled in the past 20 years. Sixteen percent of children and adolescents between 6 and 19 years old are considered overweight.

Symptoms

Consumption of more food than the body can use

Excess alcohol intake

Sedentary lifestyle

Assessing Your Risk

Three key measures are used in assessing overweight:

Body mass index (BMI)

Waist circumference

Risk factors for diseases and conditions associated with obesity

The BMI is a measure of your weight in relation to your height, and your waist circumference measures your abdominal fat. Combining these with information about your additional risk factors will give you an idea of your risk for developing obesity-associated diseases.

What is your risk?

· Body Mass Index (BMI)

BMI is a reliable indicator of total body fat, which is linked to the risk of disease and death. However, while the score is valid, it may overestimate body fat in those with a muscular build, and it may underestimate body fat in older persons or others without much muscle mass.

Use BMI tables to estimate your total body fat:

BMI below 18.5: Underweight

BMI 18.5 - 24.9: Normal

BMI 25.0 - 29.9: Overweight

BMI 30.0 and Above: Obese

· Waist circumference

Your waist circumference (which you can find by placing a measuring tape snugly around your waist) is a good indicator of your abdominal fat. This is another predictor of developing risk for heart disease and other illnesses. This risk increases with a waist measurement of over 40 inches in men and over 35 inches in women.

·Risk of obesity-associated diseases

The combination of your BMI and your waist circumference informs you of an increased risk for developing obesity-associated diseases or conditions.

Other risk factors
·Besides being overweight or obese, other risk factors are important to consider:
·High blood pressure (hypertension)
·High LDL-cholesterol ("bad" cholesterol)
·Low HDL-cholesterol ("good" cholesterol)
·High triglycerides
·High blood glucose (sugar)
·Family history of premature heart disease
·Physical inactivity
·Cigarette smoking

Assessment

For obese or overweight people who have two or more risk factors, federal guidelines recommend weight loss. Even a small weight loss (such as 10 percent of your current weight) lowers your chance of developing diseases associated with obesity. Patients who are overweight but have less than 2 risk factors and do not have a high waist measurement may just need to prevent further weight gain rather than lose weight.

Ask your doctor to evaluate your BMI, waist measurement and others risk factors for heart disease. He can let you know your level of risk and whether you should lose weight.

Causes

· Lack of physical activity

The risk of developing coronary heart disease, the nation's leading cause of death, can be significantly decreased by regular physical activity. This will also decrease the risk for colon cancer, diabetes and high blood pressure. It also helps with weight control and the development of healthy bones, muscles and joints; reduces falls among the elderly; helps to relieve arthritic pain; reduces symptoms of anxiety and depression; and is associated with fewer hospitalizations, physician visits and medications.

More than 60 percent of American adults do not get enough physical activity to provide health benefits, with more than 25 percent being virtually inactive in their leisure time. Activity decreases with age and is less common among women than men and among those with lower income and less education. Adults are not the only ones who don't get enough physical activity. More than a third of youngsters in grades 9-12 do not regularly engage in vigorous physical activity.

· The critical role of healthy eating

At least 10 million Americans at risk for Type 2 diabetes can sharply lower their chances of getting the disease with good nutrition and proper exercise. Only about one-fourth of U.S. adults eat the recommended five or more servings of fruits and vegetables daily. More than 60 percent of young people eat too much fat, and less than 20 percent eat the recommended five or more servings of fruits and vegetables each day.

Treatment

First, a person should set realistic goals for weight reduction.

Key recommendations from the expert panel on the Identification, Evaluation and Treatment of Overweight and Obesity in Adults:

The initial goal of weight-loss therapy should be to reduce body weight by about 10 percent from baseline. For the first six months, weight loss should be approximately one to two pounds per week. If necessary, the patient can continue to lose more weight. Reducing dietary fat alone without reducing calories is not enough to cause weight loss.

· *Guide to physical activity*

Not only is exercise an integral part of a weight loss and weight maintenance plan, it also reduces the risk of cardiovascular disease and diabetes, beyond that produced by weight reduction alone.

Your exercise can be done all at one time, or intermittently over the day. Initial activities may be walking or swimming at a slow pace. Your regimen can be adapted to other forms of physical activity, but walking is a particularly smart choice because of its safety and accessibility. Increasing activity by undertaking frequent, less strenuous exercises, such as walking up and down the stairs instead of the using the elevator. You may eventually be able to engage in more strenuous activities such as tennis or any form of group sport.

· *Guide to behavior change*.

Weight can affect a person's self-esteem. Excess weight is clearly visible and may attract ridicule. The amount of weight loss needed to improve your health may be much less than your total weight-loss goal. Your health can be greatly improved by a loss of 5-10 percent of your starting weight. That doesn't mean you have to stop there, but it does mean that an initial goal of losing 5-10 percent of your starting weight is both realistic and valuable.

Balance your (food) checkbook

Shop for quick low fat food items and fill your kitchen cupboards with a supply of basics like the following:

Fat free or low-fat milk, yogurt, cheese, and cottage cheese.
Light or diet margarine,
Eggs/Egg substitutes,
Sandwich breads, bagels, pita bread,
English muffins.
Soft corn tortillas, low fat flour tortillas,
Low fat, low sodium crackers,
Plain cereal, dry or cooked.
Rice, pasta,
White meat chicken or turkey (remove skin),
Fish and shellfish (not battered).
Beef: round, sirloin, chuck arm, loin and extra lean ground beef,
Pork: leg, shoulder, tenderloin,
Dry beans and peas.
Fresh, frozen, canned fruits in light syrup or juice.
Fresh, frozen, or no salt added canned vegetables.
Low fat or nonfat salad dressings,
Mustard and catsup, Jam, jelly, or honey,
Herbs and spices,
Salsa

What is Food Addiction?

Food addiction is a disorder characterized by preoccupation with food, the availability of food and the anticipation of pleasure from the ingestion of food. Food addiction involves the repetitive consumption of food against the individuals better judgment resulting in loss of control and preoccupation or the restriction of food and preoccupation with body weight and image.

Types of food addiction

Anorexia Nervosa is characterized by intense fear of gaining weight.

Behavior includes excessive weighing, excessive measuring of body parts, and persistently using a mirror to check body size. Self-esteem is dependent upon body shape and weight. Weight loss is viewed as an impressive achievement and an example of extraordinary self discipline.

Physical implications may include disruption of the menstrual cycle, signs of starvation, thinning of hair or hair loss, bloated feeling, yellowish palms/soles of feet, dry, pasty skin.

Bulimia Nervosa is described as binge eating and compensatory behavior to prevent weight gain. Individuals become ashamed of their eating behavior and attempt to conceal symptoms through rapid consumption of food. They will eat until painfully full and stop if intruded upon.

80-90% of bulimics will induce vomiting. Other behaviors include, misuse of laxatives, fasting and excessive exercise.

Physical implications include, loss of dental enamel, increase of cavities, swollen saliva glands, calluses, scars on hands, irregular menstrual cycle, dependency on laxatives for bowel movements, fluid and electrolyte disturbance.

Compulsive Overeaters use food inappropriately and eventually become addicted to it and lose control over the amount of food they eat. Overeaters demonstrate uncontrollable binge eating without extreme weight control and see that behavior as normal.

Overeaters present with moderate to severe obesity, with an average binge eater being 60% overweight. Bingeing episodes consist of carbohydrates and junk food with most binges done in scheduled secrecy.

These resources can provide for you some crucial although painful facts about your struggle. Sometimes the hardest part of doing this research is being told the truth. I have found that my lifestyle left much to be desired.

I have gathered these facts to help both of us in our battle. So take down these sites and do some research on your own. Use this information as a weapon in your fight.

RESOURCES:
Center for Disease Control
National Heart, Lung and Blood Institute
National Institutes of Health - National Library of Medicine
U.S. Department of Health and Human Services
National Institute of Diabetes & Digestive & Kidney Diseases.
www.wrongdiagnosis.com/medical/obesity.htm
http://www.psychologytoday.com/conditions/obesity.html
http://www.addictionrecov.org/foodwhat.htm

DIET IDEAS

In this next chapter I am going to lay out some of my own ideas for a diet plan. Now I hope that you will remember that I suggested that you find a licensed dietician to help you plan out your correct diet. Each person has a unique metabolic rate and their diet needs to be fashioned according to that rate. Therefore understand that this diet plan and the two that I will also provide for you are only suggestions.

The correct diet (as stated earlier) should consist of a low calorie, low sugar, high protein diet. Each meal should be balanced and each diet should include exercise, and a daily vitamin supplement.

Please only consider these diet plans as suggestions and consult a dietician and your personal physician before beginning any diet or exercise regimen.

This diet plan is the first in my original book. It is eight meals that are based on a low calorie intake, high protein diet with daily exercise.

The key to finding the right diet plan for your self is to listen to what your body tells you. Know your limitations. Know your weaknesses. This means to also know your cravings.

So many dieters try to overcome their own personal cravings all at one time. They go into their diet **"cold turkey"**. The problem with this approach is that it is destined to fail. You will come across that one particular compulsion that you have and fall hard. The next step is to just give up.

The best way to overcome these areas of your diet is to know what you have cravings for. Many of these cravings are your body's way of telling you that you are low in certain minerals. Some times it is just your body's way of self-medicating. You may be under stress and you feel a craving for chocolate. This may be a way that your body has found to self-medicate.

Knowing your own weakness is your weapon in this battle. You can plan a splurge day. This means that you give yourself one day a week that you are allowed to splurge. You can plan that day to have your chocolate or cheese cake.

This allows you that freedom. Now don't be foolish and binge on that day but know that you can satisfy your craving.

Now depending on your goal you will need to customize your diet to meet that goal. The following is an article in bodybuilding.com by one of their sports nutritionists. This diet is designed for the average bodybuilder or beginner bodybuilder but it does give some vital information concerning diet and proper nutrition.

I have tried to summarize most of the information for lack of space and overload of information. So please understand this as you read through the information that if you wish to read the whole article please go to the web site mentioned and you can get all the information.

"Before getting to the actual diet, there are many things that need to be covered. The mechanisms behind successful fat loss are just as important as the diet itself. By understanding these, you will be able to tell which diet plans will work well, and why other diet plans which seem to be good, are not really that great at all.

As there is no single diet that is best for everyone, you will be better able to adjust a diet plan after reading these things.

There are many common mistakes that can hinder fat loss results.

Under-eating: Not consuming enough food, or enough of the right foods will hinder your fat loss goals in many ways. The fewer calories you consume, the more efficient your metabolism becomes. In most cases, efficiency is a good thing. In this case, it is not. If calories levels are too low, your muscle tissue stands a much bigger chance of being burned for energy. Decreased calories can also significantly reduce performance in the gym.

Over-eating: Eating too many calories, or too much of the wrong foods is just as bad. On one hand, eating more will cause your body to burn more total calories, and will make your metabolism more inefficient. However, this is a tool which must be used intelligently; it does not mean you can eat as much as you want.

Not Eating Frequently Enough: Nearly every bodybuilder understands on some level that eating smaller, more frequent meals is important.

The first, and most well known reason is to provide the body with a steady supply of protein. Maintaining a supply of protein is crucial for building muscle, and it is very important for fat loss & preventing muscle loss as well. The body cannot store protein for future use, so providing a steady stream of amino acids is extremely important.

The next reason involves hourly energy balance. Eating frequently is important for providing your body with just enough nutrients it needs at that given moment.

Thinking In Terms Of 24-Hour Energy Balance: Too many people think in calories per day, total carbs per day, or grams of protein per day. Your body however, does not share this same though process. When you consume food at any time, your body will use what it can, and store the rest as fat.

A large portion of those ends up being stored as fat.. Later on, when their body needs, and can use carbohydrates, less are consumed. Glycogen stores do not get replenished to the same degree. Some protein ends up being burned as energy, because sufficient carbs were not available at that moment.

At the end of the day, weight was lost, because calories burned exceeded calories eaten. However, extra muscle tissue was lost, and less fat was burned. Possibly little to no fat may have been burned. Moment-to-moment, or hourly energy balance is much more important that daily energy balance.

Not Paying Attention To Meal & Nutrient Timing:

As mentioned before, the amount of food consumed at any particular time is an important concept. Similar to calorie needs at any given moment, the body has specific needs for certain macronutrients at any given movement.

Protein is needed just about all the time, but there are times when even more of it is needed. Not paying attention to this, and thinking that you are good to go just because you met your macro. Quotas, is another mistake.

Consuming Too Few Carbohydrates: Very low carb, or ketogenic diets are a fairly popular method of weight loss. While people do get results with these types of diets, they are neither necessary, nor ideal for fat loss.

Carbohydrates are crucial for ideal performance in the gym. Having optimum performance is very important for losing fat. Having a certain level of carbohydrates in the body is also important for sparing muscle tissue from catabolism. A slight reduction of carbs can be beneficial. Carb cycling can be an excellent method, if used intelligently. But drastically reducing carbs yields many more drawbacks than possible benefits.

Not Consuming Enough Fats: Even people who understand the importance of fats in the diet sometimes unknowingly reduce fats way too much when cutting. Therefore, it is important to pay special attention to fat intake to ensure that you are getting the optimal quantity and types of fat.

Fats are essential for the production of nearly every hormone, including testosterone. They are important for metabolic function, skin health, immune health, and many other things. Essential fatty acids, especially omega-3 fatty acids, are largely responsible for many of these benefits. Fish oil, which contains the omega-3 acids DHA and EPA, can provide some outstanding benefits for anyone trying to get the best possible body for summertime. More information on that will be given later.

Not Drinking Enough Water:

It would be hard to find a bodybuilder who did not know the importance of consuming sufficient amounts of water. However, it would be rather easy to find one who did not actually consume enough.

When effort is not made to drink enough water, it is easy to fall far short of the optimal amount. The biggest reason this happens comes from relying on thirst. In many people, the thirst mechanism is not a reliable measure of when water is needed. As a general rule, your urine should stay clear or a very light yellow. If it starts to significantly darken, it could be a sign of dehydration.

The Macronutrients:

Here we will briefly cover the macronutrients, their role in the body, and basic consumption guidelines.

Protein:

Proteins are made up of amino acids, and are used to build nearly every tissue in the body, including muscle. There are 20 main amino acids, 10 of which are essential amino acids.

Essential aminos are ones that cannot be synthesized from other amino acids, and must be supplied in the diet. Therefore, if you are lacking in just 1 essential amino acids, results can be hindered. To ensure that you get all necessary amino acids, consume a variety of protein sources, ideally with one of those being from meat.

Approximately 1 gram of protein per pound of bodyweight is plenty for nearly everyone. For a 200 lb person, this is 200 grams of protein. With proper nutrient timing, muscle mass can often be built with less. However, slightly higher protein intake offers further benefits for fat loss, including hormonal benefits, increased thermic effect, and better maintenance of muscle mass while on a diet.

Good Protein Sources: Eggs, Fish, Lean red meats, Poultry, Low-fat or Fat-free or raw milk, Whey, Casein

Carbohydrates:

Carbohydrates are the prime source of fuel for exercise, as well as for the brain and nervous system. Carbohydrates are used to replenish glycogen stores, which is important for providing the body with a store of glucose.

Optimally maintaining glycogen stores are important for sparing muscle proteins from breakdown, as well as optimizing performance in the gym. Aim to consume 30%-50% of your calories from carbohydrates.

Good Carbohydrate Sources: Whole grains, Oats, Fruits, Fibrous vegetables, Starchy vegetables, Whole grain pastas or breads, Sprouted breads

Fats:

Fatty acids are an essential nutrient in the body. With regards to fat loss, they are especially important for hormonal production, including testosterone and thyroid hormones. They also play roles in protein synthesis, immune system health, skin health, joint health, and much more.

Ideally, one should consume most of their fats from certain polyunsaturated and monounsaturated sources. Some of the fats can come from saturated sources, but ideally limit this to one-third or less of total fat intake. Aim to consume 20-30% of calories from fats, most of which are non-animal sources.

Good Fat Sources: Fish oil, Flax seeds & oil, Olive oil, **Fish, Nuts, Coconut oil, Avocados**

It can be hard to consume all of your fats from these sources. Eggs & lean meats are ok as a source of fat, but make sure that these make up the smaller, rather than the larger share of your fat intake.

Hormones That Influence Fat Loss:

Testosterone levels are important for building & maintaining muscle, as well as influencing fat loss. You can help to maintain ideal levels by consuming sufficient fats, getting enough rest, and by using certain nutritional supplements which will be discussed later.

Insulin is a double-edged sword. It is essential for protein synthesis and facilitating the uptake up nutrients into muscle cells, among many other things.

High levels at certain times are desirable. A low/moderate, constant level is desirable most of the time.

On the other hand, high levels at the wrong times can lead to increased fat storage. Nutrient timing is key to having optimal levels of insulin at the right times.

Cortisol is a catabolic hormone which helps to break down fat and muscle into glucose. High levels trigger muscle breakdown much more than fat. Certain levels are necessary for health & balance.

High levels can be triggered by physical stress (after intense exercise), or by psychological stress.

Glucagon is a catabolic hormone which triggers liver glycogen breakdown, and in come cases, protein breakdown. It can also stimulate the breakdown of lipolysis (fat breakdown). The regular consumption of protein can raise glucagon levels. Maintaining glycogen stores is an important part of minimizing protein conversion into glucose.

Post Workout Nutrition is perhaps the most important meal of the day. The timing of it is very important as well. Delaying post workout nutrition by even 30 minutes can significantly reduce its benefits. It is important to consume both carbohydrates and protein as soon as possible after a workout.

As you can see, it is important that the nutrient get to the muscle cells as soon as possible. So obviously, we want fast absorbing & fast digesting nutrients. For this reason, liquid meals are ideal. Fast absorbing carbohydrates are also ideal.

Maltodextrin is probably the best source, as it is absorbed by the stomach faster than sucrose or dextrose. Whey is the ideal choice for a protein source. 1-2 grams of extra glutamine and BCAA's are also very beneficial. Aim to consume about 30 grams of protein, and 60-80 grams of carbohydrate, or .25 g/lb of protein, and .5 -.75 g/lb of carbohydrate.

Before Bed Nutrition: While this is more important for building muscle, it is also important for a fat loss diet, as it will greatly help to reduce possible muscle loss. Pre-bed meals should be mostly protein, with a very small amount of carbohydrate, and possibly a very small amount of fat.

The protein source should be a mix of fast absorbing & slow absorbing protein. Whey powder mixed with casein and skim milk is perfect for a bedtime shake. This shake should be lower in overall calories than a post workout shake.

Eat More To Burn More: When most people calculate their cutting diet, they subtract a certain amount from what they think is their maintenance level of calories. The body's metabolic rate constantly changes. When you eat more, especially when those foods are ideal food choices & eaten at the right times, the body's metabolism greatly increases.

The body becomes more inefficient, and wastes more calories as heat with all of its metabolic processes. Eating a lot of low-calorie fruits and vegetables is a great way to boost this. By eating more, you burn more total calories, and more fat is burned as a result.

Cheat Meals:

A cheat meal once per week is perfectly acceptable. It is important, though, to cheat with food types, rather than excess calories. This means that you can have some chips, some sweets, or some beer. But you still need to stay within the same calorie ranges. Binging with 4000 extra calories of junk food can cancel out several days-worth of hard work.

However, if you do not feel the need, or do not want to eat cheat foods, then it is fine to stay on your diet 7 days per week. Any benefits of a cheat meal are 100% psychological, although those benefits can be substantial.

Fruits & Vegetables:

The fruits and vegetables listed can, and should be eaten frequently (barring pre and post workout). The ones listed do not need to be counted towards total calories or carbohydrates. I am sure some of you reading this are screaming "Of course they do!!!" However, the reason for this has to do with the concept of metabolic flux, a highly modifiable metabolism & the high thermogenic effect of these foods.

Fruits: Grapefruits , Watermelon , Strawberries, Blackberries, Currants, Blueberries, Rhubarb, Oranges, Cantaloupe

Vegetables: All fibrous, low-calorie vegetables. These are vegetables such as: Carrots, Celery, Lettuce, Other leafy greens, Cucumbers, Turnips, Tomatoes, Radishes, Broccoli ,Cauliflower"

In this chapter I have given you an abundance of information and I want to close out this chapter with a diet plan that has worked for me. Use this as a simple guide. Remember as I said before that all I am doing is assisting you in finding the answers. So in this table I have laid out each meal and also a series of supplements that are helpful.

Always use the rule of not eating two hours before bed time. This will allow the body to burn fat during the night. Many people suffer from insomnia or night cravings and this is one of the reasons for this problem.

If you desire more information please check out the last chapter and you will be able to get more information from the bodybuilding.com web page. In this information you will see a calculation for BMR and Macronutrient Ratios, as well as a diet plan.

Sunday	Monday	Tuesday	Wednesday	Thursday	Friday	Saturday
Breakfast	Breakfast	Breakfast	Breakfast	Breakfast	Breakfast	Breakfast
Oatmeal	Oatmeal	Oatmeal	Oatmeal	Oatmeal	Oatmeal	Oatmeal
Mid-Am Meal	*Mid-Am Meal*	*Mid-Am Meal*	*Mid-Am Meal*	*Mid-Am Meal*	*Mid-Am Meal*	*Mid-Am Meal*
Bowl of fruit/ Diet shake	Bowl of fruit/ Diet Shake/ Eggs	Bowl of fruit/ Diet shake	Bowl of fruit/ Diet Shake/ Eggs	Bowl of fruit/ Diet shake	Bowl of fruit/ Diet Shake/ Eggs	Bowl of fruit/ Diet shake
Lunch	*Lunch*	*Lunch*	*Lunch*	*Lunch*	*Lunch*	*Lunch*
Diet Shake/ Salad/ Chicken/ Wheat Toast	Salad/ Fish/ Diet shake/ Muffin	Diet Shake/ Salad/ Chicken/ Wheat Toast	Diet Shake/ Salad/ Chicken/ Wheat Toast	Salad/ Fish/ Diet shake/ Muffin	Diet Shake/ Salad/ Chicken/ Wheat Toast	Salad/ Fish/ Diet shake/ Muffin
Late-Am Meal	*Late-Am Meal*	*Late-Am Meal*	*Late-Am Meal*	*Late-Am Meal*	*Late-Am Meal*	*Late-Am Meal*
Fruit/ Diet Shake/ Salad	Fruit/ Diet Shake/ Salad	Fruit/ Diet Shake/ Salad	Fruit/ Diet Shake/ Salad	Fruit/ Diet Shake/ Salad	Fruit/ Diet Shake/ Salad	Fruit/ Diet Shake/ Salad
Dinner	*Dinner*	*Dinner*	*Dinner*	*Dinner*	*Dinner*	*Dinner*
Steak/ Veggies/ Soup/ Diet Shake	Chicken/ Salad/Muffin / Diet Shake	Fish Veggies/ Diet Shake	Steak/ Veggies/ soup Diet Shake	Chicken/ Salad/muffin / Diet Shake	Fish Veggies/ Diet Shake	Steak/ Salad/ Veggies/ Diet Shake
Late Evening	*Late Evening*	*Late Evening*	*Late Evening*	*Late Evening*	*Late Evening*	*Late Evening*
Diet Shake	Diet Shake	Diet Shake	Diet Shake	Diet Shake	Diet Shake	Diet Shake

Sunday	Monday	Tuesday	Wednesday	Thursday	Friday	Saturday
Breakfast	*Breakfast*	*Breakfast*	*Breakfast*	*Breakfast*	*Breakfast*	*Breakfast*
Diet Shake	Diet Shake	Diet Shake	Diet Shake	Diet Shake	Diet Shake	Diet Shake
Mid-Am Meal	*Mid-Am Meal*	*Mid-Am Meal*	*Mid-Am Meal*	*Mid-Am Meal*	*Mid-Am Meal*	*Mid-Am Meal*
Oatmeal/ Fruit/ Diet Shake	Eggs/ Diet Shake	Eggs/ Diet Shake	Oatmeal/ Fruit/ Diet Shake	Eggs/ Diet Shake	Eggs/ Diet Shake	Oatmeal/ Fruit/ Diet Shake
Lunch	*Lunch*	*Lunch*	*Lunch*	*Lunch*	*Lunch*	*Lunch*
Salad/ Chicken/ Veggies/ Diet Shake	Salad/ Fruit/ Diet Shake	Salad/ Fruit/ Diet Shake	Salad/ Chicken/ Veggies/ Diet Shake	Salad/ Fruit/ Diet Shake	Salad/ Fruit/ Diet Shake	Salad/ Chicken/ Veggies/ Diet Shake
Late-Am Meal	*Late-Am Meal*	*Late-Am Meal*	*Late-Am Meal*	*Late-Am Meal*	*Late-Am Meal*	*Late-Am Meal*
Fruit/ Diet Shake	Fruit/ Diet Shake	Fruit/ Diet Shake	Fruit/ Diet Shake	Fruit/ Diet Shake	Fruit/ Diet Shake	Fruit/ Diet Shake
Dinner	*Dinner*	*Dinner*	*Dinner*	*Dinner*	*Dinner*	*Dinner*
Steak/ Salad/ Veggies/ Diet Shake	Steak/ Salad/ Diet Shake	Steak/ Salad/ Diet Shake	Steak/ Salad/ Veggies/ Diet Shake	Steak/ Salad/ Diet Shake	Steak/ Salad/ Diet Shake	Steak/ Salad/ Veggies/ Diet Shake
Late Evening	*Late Evening*	*Late Evening*	*Late Evening*	*Late Evening*	*Late Evening*	*Late Evening*
Diet Shake	Diet Shake	Diet Shake	Diet Shake	Diet Shake	Diet Shake	Diet Shake

EXERCISE PLANS

The exercise plan is a vital part of your diet program. Too often people attempt to loose weight and fail to add a solid exercise plan into their daily life. This is a failure waiting to happen. Diet needs to be accompanied with an exercise program. The body needs to have a complete change in it's metabolic rate.

Often we fail to even try to start an exercise program because of embarrassment or simply laziness. The truth is that any form of movement that will bring your body temp and heart rate up is sufficient. A daily walk, or even simply doing sit-ups or push-ups during the day will produce the results that you need.

Reality is that many of us are obese to the point that we need to use extreme caution when attempting this activity. Please contact your physician before attempting any activity and monitor how your body reacts to this. You know your body and you will know when something is not right.

If you are unable to do push-ups then simply lean into the wall and push away from the wall. Attempt at least ten of these and then set a goal to continue this each night until you can do twenty. With each attempt try to lower the height that you are working from. When you can, use a chair to lean against . Keep a record and try to monitor our success.

Walking should be at a steady pace that will bring your heart rate up to a steady level. able to carry on a conversation without being completely out of breath.

What ever you attempt keep doing this and keep it to only thirty minutes. Eventually you will reach a point that you can actually go into a gym. At this point contact a trainer and tell him/her the goals that you have set for yourself. Don't be shy. Tell him/her that you want to be able to put on a nice swim suit and not be ashamed to go to the beach.

My personal goal is that I want to be able to stand on a stage and do a pose down in a bodybuilding competition. I don't really care if I win or lose. This is what I have set for myself and I will reach that goal. So be looking for the Miracle Body that was once over 400lbs.

But enough talk. Let me show you the basic plan that I used to work out. It isn't that difficult to follow. If you maintain a steady workout with a minimum of four days a week, you can reach your goal rather easily.

I am going to first lay out some specific exercises and how to do them without hurting yourself. The first main principle is to always drink a lot of water and to stretch. Stretching is the main component to avoiding injury when you do any type of exercise. Stretching loosens the muscles and tendons to prepare them for strenuous work.

Keep this in mind as you look at the proper lifting methods for each exercise. I have included some of the lifts that are specifically for those who are wanting to put on mass and some lifts for those trying to work on strength and endurance.

This workout is designed for a beginner bodybuilder. It is a preparation for an increasingly intense workout plan. The plan for this workout is to do the three and twenty for three weeks and then change to a mass building workout.

The following would be a standard mass building workout that I would use. Understand that I am working toward a goal of competition so your personal work out may be extremely different than this.

What you are going to be seeing in this type of workout program is a pyramid system. This is designed where with each set you will increase your weight by five to ten pounds. You are not wanting to have a rep of more than eight to ten. This will maintain your burn.

Understanding that this workout is designed for a little more intense individual than you can adjust this to meet your specific goals. Overall it is a great general workout program and can work with the beginner or the more experienced individual.

I have decided to also include the following group of exercises from my favorite web site, "bodybuilding.com". This is valuable information because it also includes photos demonstrating the proper form and tips on how to get the best from each lift.

Please check out each lift and how to do them correctly. I have also added stretches and warm ups so you can avoid any chance of injury.

MONDAY: BACK WK 1	
DEADLIFTS	Three sets/ min. 20 reps
LOW ROW	Three sets/ min. 20 reps
BAR SHRUGS	Three sets/ min. 20 reps
LAT PULL DOWN	Three sets/ min. 20 reps
STIFF DEAD LIFTS	Three sets/ min. 20 reps

TUESDAY: CHEST WK 1	
FLAT BENCH	Three sets/ min. 20 reps
INCLINE BENCH	Three sets/ min. 20 reps
CLOSE GRIP	Three sets/ min. 20 reps
INCLINE DUMB BELL	Three sets/ min. 20 reps
MACHINE PRESS	Three sets/ min. 20 reps

WEDNESDAY: ARMS WK 1	
SKULL CRUSHERS	Three sets/ min. 20 reps
TRICEP PRES	Three sets/ min. 20 reps
ONE ARM REVERSE GRIP	Three sets/ min. 20 reps
LYING HAMMER	Three sets/ min. 20 reps
BAR CURLS	Three sets/ min. 20 reps
HAMMER CURLS	Three sets/ min. 20 reps
CABLE CURLS	Three sets/ min. 20 reps
CONCENTRATION CURLS	Three sets/ min. 20 reps

THURSDAY: LEGS WK	
SQUATS	Three sets/ min. 20 reps
LEG PRESS	Three sets/ min. 20 reps
LEG EXTENSIONS	Three sets/ min. 20 reps
LEG CURLS	Three sets/ min. 20 reps
ABDUCTION	Three sets/ min. 20 reps
ADDUCTION	Three sets/ min. 20 reps

FRIDAY: SHOULDERS/ TRAPS WK 1	
SEATED FRONT RAISE	Three sets/ min. 20 reps
SEATED SIDE RAISE	Three sets/ min. 20 reps
SEATED DB PRESS	Three sets/ min. 20 reps
REVERSE DELT RAISE	Three sets/ min. 20 reps
SHOULDER PRESS	Three sets/ min. 20 reps

SATUERDAY: ABS/CALFS WK 1	
CABLE CRUNCH	Three sets/ min. 20 reps
AB MACHINE	Three sets/ min. 20 reps
INCLINE SIT UP	Three sets/ min. 20 reps
LYING CRUNCH	Three sets/ min. 20 reps
CALF PRESS	Three sets/ min. 20 reps
SEATED CALF RAISE	Three sets/ min. 20 reps

MONDAY: CHEST/ ABS WK 4					
LIFT	REPETITIONS				
CRUNCH	25	25	15	15	10
FLAT BENCH	15	8-10	8-10	8-10	8-10
INCLINE	15	8-10	8-10	8-10	8-10
DECLINE	15	8-10	8-10	8-10	8-10
D'BELL FLAT	15	8-10	8-10	8-10	8-10
D'BELL N'CLINE	15	8-10	8-10	8-10	8-10
PEC MACHINE	15	8-10	8-10	8-10	8-10
CABLE CROSS	15	8-10	8-10	8-10	8-10
AB MACHINE	15	8-10	8-10	8-10	8-10
TUESDAY: QUADS/ HAMS/ CALVES WK 4					
LIFTS	REPETITIONS				
LEG EXTENSIONS	25	25	15	15	10
LOW CABLE ROW	15	8-10	8-10	8-10	8-10
LEG PRESS	15	8-10	8-10	8-10	8-10
LEG CURLS	15	8-10	8-10	8-10	8-10
CALF PRESS	15	8-10	8-10	8-10	8-10
SEATED CALF	15	8-10	8-10	8-10	8-10
DEAD LIFTS	15	8-10	8-10	8-10	8-10
ABDUCTION	15	8-10	8-10	8-10	8-10
ADDUCTION	15	8-10	8-10	8-10	8-10
AB MACHINE	15	8-10	8-10	8-10	8-10
WEDNESDAY: SHOULDERS/ TRAPS/ ABS WK					
LIFTS	REPETITIONS				
BENT LAT D'BELL	25	25	15	15	10
D'BELL LAT RAISE	15	8-10	8-10	8-10	8-10
D'BELL FT RAISE	15	8-10	8-10	8-10	8-10
D'BELL SHOULDER	15	8-10	8-10	8-10	8-10
WIDE CABLE ROW	15	8-10	8-10	8-10	8-10
BAR SHRUGS	15	8-10	8-10	8-10	8-10
SHOULDER PRESS	15	8-10	8-10	8-10	8-10
DELT RAISE	15	8-10	8-10	8-10	8-10
REVERSE DELT	15	8-10	8-10	8-10	8-10
LAT MACHINE	15	8-10	8-10	8-10	8-10
CRUNCH	15	8-10	8-10	8-10	8-10
AB MACHINE	15	8-10	8-10	8-10	8-10

THURSDAY: ARMS/ FORARMS WK 4					
LIFTS	REPETITIONS				
TRICEP CABLE	25	25	15	15	10
CLOSE GRIP BENCH	15	8-10	8-10	8-10	8-10
TRICEP MACHINE	15	8-10	8-10	8-10	8-10
BICEP MACHINE	15	8-10	8-10	8-10	8-10
BAR CURLS	15	8-10	8-10	8-10	8-10
CONCENTRATION	15	8-10	8-10	8-10	8-10
BAR WRIST	15	8-10	8-10	8-10	8-10
BAR REVERSE	15	8-10	8-10	8-10	8-10
BAR CABLE	15	8-10	8-10	8-10	8-10
FRIDAY: B ACK AND CALF:WK 4					
LIFTS	REPETITIONS				
BENT SMITH ROW	25	25	15	15	10
STIFF-ARM PULL	15	8-10	8-10	8-10	8-10
ONE ARM ROWS	15	8-10	8-10	8-10	8-10
LAT MACHINE	15	8-10	8-10	8-10	8-10
REVERSE LAT	15	8-10	8-10	8-10	8-10
CALF PRESS	15	8-10	8-10	8-10	8-10
SEATED CALF PRESS	15	8-10	8-10	8-10	8-10
BACK BENCH	15	8-10	8-10	8-10	8-10
DEAD LIFT	15	8-10	8-10	8-10	8-10
BACK MACHINE	15	8-10	8-10	8-10	8-10
SATURDAY: CARDIO WK 4					
LIFTS	REPETITIONS				
TREADMILL	25	25	15	15	10
CABLE TWIST	15	8-10	8-10	8-10	8-10
LEG RAISE	15	8-10	8-10	8-10	8-10
CRUNCHES	15	8-10	8-10	8-10	8-10
HEAVY BAG	15	8-10	8-10	8-10	8-10
STATIONARY BIKE	15	8-10	8-10	8-10	8-10
AB MACHINE	15	8-10	8-10	8-10	8-10
BACK MACHINE	15	8-10	8-10	8-10	8-10

Barbell Dead lift
Exercise Data
Main Muscle Worked: Quadriceps.

Other Muscles Worked: Hamstrings, Calves, Glutes.

Equipment: Barbell.

Mechanics Type: Compound .

Tips: Think of a dead lift as a squat, only the bar is in your hands rather than on your back.

The Stance: Approach the loaded barbell and assume a stance about as wide as your own shoulders while gripping the bar such that the inner aspects of your arms are slightly outside of your thighs. Another way to determine your optimal dead lift foot placement is to jump down from a box which is half your own height and "stick" the landing. Now look at your feet...this will approximate your ideal stance width and degree of foot turn-out.

Feet and Shin Position: Feet should point straight forward or turned out to a 25 degree angle at most. The best foot angle is one which provides the least amount of hip and knee restriction when you lower the hips in preparation to lift, so don't be afraid to experiment a bit. The shins should be two to three inches from the bar and then when you actually bend down and lower your hips in preparation to lift, the shins will touch the bar. Most of the weight will be on the heels of the feet. This facilitates maximal contribution of the glutes and hamstrings. During the ascent, the bar will travel as close to the leg and shins as possible. Ideally, wear cotton sweat pants or track pants with long socks to protect your shins.

Hand Position: A "reverse grip" should be used when dead lifting. This means that one hand will be supinated (palm faces you) and the other pronated (palm facing away). This will help keep the bar in your hand. If grip strength is not one of your training targets, feel free to use wrist straps with a conventional grip. Hold the bar high up on the palm to compensate for any roll of the bar when pulling the weight up. Generally, the grip should start with the index finger and the little finger bordering the knurling in the middle of the bar.

Head Placement and Eye Contact: The entire spine should remain neutral, which means you look neither up nor down, but instead, the head follows the body, almost like you're wearing a cervical cast on your neck. It's OK for the head to be SLIGHTLY up (this tends to improve muscular contraction of the low back muscles) but in all cases, the lift must start with the hips down, the entire spine neutral, and the feet flat on the floor.

The Ascent: As you stand up with the weight, imagine pushing the earth away from you with your feet. When viewed from the side, your hips and shoulders should ascend together; if the hips rise before the shoulders, it means you're using your back rather than your legs. If this happens, reduce the weight until you can perform the lift correctly and add more specific quad-strengthening exercises to your program.

The Lockout: Competitive power lifters are required to demonstrate control over the weight by standing up and then extending the hips forward in an exaggerated manner. If you're NOT a competitive lifter, simply stand up with the weight without this exaggerated maneuver.

The Descent: Simply return the bar to the floor, under control, by reversing the technique you used to lift the weight.

The Wrong Way:

Elevated Cable Rows
Exercise Data
Main Muscle Worked: Lats
Other Muscles Worked: Middle Back
Equipment: Cable
Mechanics Type: Compound

Tips: Get a platform of some sort that is around 4-6" in height (calf raise platform, aerobics platform etc). Place it on the seat of the cable row machine. Lean forward with a strong arch in your back. Keep this leaned forward position while pulling into your abs. This exercise hits the lower lats hard.

Lying T-Bar Row
Exercise Data
Main Muscle Worked: Middle Back
Other Muscles Worked: Biceps, Lats
Equipment: Machine
Mechanics Type: Compound

Tips: Adjust the leg height so that your upper chest is at the top of the pad. Lay face down on the pad and grab the handles. You can use a palms down, palms up, or palms in position depending on what part of your back you want to work more. Extend your arms completely to start. Slowly pull the weight up and squeeze your back at the top of the movement. Do not lift your body off of the pad! Return to the starting position.

Barbell Shrug
Exercise Data
Main Muscle Worked: Traps
Other Muscles Worked: None
Equipment: Barbell
Mechanics Type: Isolation

Tips: Hold a barbell with both hands in front of you with your hands a little wider than shoulder width apart. Keep your feet at shoulder width. Stand straight up with the bar hanging at arms length. Droop shoulders down as much as possible to start. Raise your shoulders up as far as you can go. You can also rotate your shoulders as you go up, going in a semicircular motion from front to rear. Then slowly return to the starting position. Can also be down with dumbbells.

Barbell Shrug Behind The Back
Exercise Data
Main Muscle Worked: Traps
Other Muscles Worked: None
Equipment: Barbell
Mechanics Type: Isolation

Tips: Hold a barbell behind your back with your palms facing backwards. "Shrug" your shoulders upward as high as you can and squeeze it for a second. Then lower the bar all the way down as far as you can. To get the barbell into position, you can rest it on a power rack or bench and then pick it up from there. You can also do these with dumbbells.

Close-Grip Front Lat Pulldown
Exercise Data
Main Muscle Worked: Lats
Other Muscles Worked: Biceps, Middle Back

Equipment: Cable
Mechanics Type: Compound
   Tips: Works the lower lats. Sit at a lat pulldown machine or kneel in front of a cable pulley. Hold lat bar with hands about 8 inches apart. Start with arms extended overhead. Pull bar straight down until it is even with your upper chest. Return slowly to starting position. Do not swing or lean back!

Stiff-Legged Dumbbell Deadlift
Exercise Data
Main Muscle Worked: Lower Back
Other Muscles Worked: Hamstrings
Equipment: Dumbbell
Mechanics Type: Compound
   Tips: Bend at your waist with your head up, back straight and knees nearly locked. Hold dumbbells at arm's length with palms facing in. Straighten up while holding the dumbbells at arm's length. Lower back down to the floor. This can be a dangerous exercise if not done correctly or done with weights that are too heavy. Can also be done standing on a bench or box or with a barbell.

Barbell Bench Press - Medium Grip
Exercise Data
Main Muscle Worked: Chest
Other Muscles Worked: Triceps, Shoulders
Equipment: Barbell
Mechanics Type: Compound
   Tips: Lie on a flat bench and firmly position your feet flat on the floor a little more than shoulder width apart. Keep your back flat on the bench! Using a grip broader than shoulder width, hold the barbell above your body, then lower slowly to the middle of your chest. Without bouncing the weight off your chest, drive the barbell up over the middle of your chest until your arms are straight and your elbows are locked. Lower the bar down slowly.

Barbell Guillotine Bench Press
Exercise Data
Main Muscle Worked: Chest

Other Muscles Worked: Triceps
Equipment: Barbell
Mechanics Type: Compound
Tips:
Preparation: Lie Horizontal on bench. Lift barbell from rack over the upper chest using a wide overhand grip. **Execution:** Lower weight to neck. Upper arms will be perpendicular to the torso. Press the bar until arms are fully extended. Repeat.

Incline Dumbbell Press
Exercise Data
Main Muscle Worked: Chest
Other Muscles Worked: Triceps, Shoulders
Equipment: Dumbbell
Mechanics Type: Compound
Tips: Sit on the edge of an incline bench set at about a 45-degree angle. Pick up a dumbbell in each hand and place them on your thighs. Then, one at a time, raise them up to your shoulder level while you press your back and shoulders firmly against the bench. Press the weights back up to a point over your upper chest, with your palms facing forward. Lower the weights slowly. Inhale as you lower the weights and exhale as you lift.

Incline Dumbbell Bench With Palms Facing In
Exercise Data
Main Muscle Worked: Chest
Other Muscles Worked: Triceps, Shoulders
Equipment: Dumbbell
Mechanics Type: Compound
Tips: Same as the Incline Dumbbell Press but with your palms facing towards each other at all times. Keep your arms close to your sides.

Barbell Incline Bench Press - Medium Grip
Exercise Data
Main Muscle Worked: Chest
Other Muscles Worked: Triceps, Shoulders

Equipment: Barbell
Mechanics Type: Compound
   Tips: Set the incline bench at about a 45 degree angle. Sit on the bench with your feet flat on the floor a little more than shoulder width apart. Position your back firmly against the bench. Using a grip slightly wider than shoulder width, hold the bar over your upper chest with your arms straight. Slowly lower the bar and make slight contact with your upper chest area. Drive the weight straight up over your chest until your elbows are locked, or close to it.

Close-Grip Barbell Bench Press
Exercise Data
Main Muscle Worked: Chest
Other Muscles Worked: Triceps, Shoulders
Equipment: Barbell
Mechanics Type: Compound
   Tips: Just like the Barbell Bench Press but with your hands only 12 - 14" apart, centered over your body. Works more of the inner pectorals and triceps.

Lying Triceps Press
Exercise Data
Main Muscle Worked: Triceps
Other Muscles Worked: None
Equipment: Barbell
Mechanics Type: Isolation
   Tips: Sit on a flat bench holding an EZ-Curl bar with an overhand grip. Lie back so that the top of your head is even with the end of the bench. At the same time, extend your arms over your head so that the bar is directly over your eyes. Keep your elbows tight and your upper arms stationary throughout the exercise. Holding your upper arms in a fixed position (this is key), slowly lower the bar until it almost touches your forehead. Then press the bar back up in a slow, sweeping arc-like motion. At the finish, lock your elbows completely.

Standing Overhead Barbell Triceps Extension
Exercise Data
Main Muscle Worked: Triceps

Other Muscles Worked: None
Equipment: Barbell
Mechanics Type: Isolation
   Tips: Hold barbell or EZ Curl bar with hands about 6 to 8 inches apart. Raise bar overhead to arm's length. Lower bar in a semicircular motion behind head until your forearms touch your biceps. Keep your upper arms close to your head. Do not move your elbows! Return to starting position. Can also be done seated.

Lying Close-Grip Barbell Triceps Press To Chin
Exercise Data
Main Muscle Worked: Triceps
Other Muscles Worked: None
Equipment: Barbell
Mechanics Type: Isolation
   Tips: Lie on your back on a flat bench with your head off the end. Hold a barbell or EZ Curl bar with hands about 6 inches apart. Press bar to your arm's length above your shoulders. Lower bar in a semicircular motion to chin, bending arms at your elbows, keeping your upper arms vertical. Return to starting position. Never move your elbows!

Cable One Arm Tricep Extension
Exercise Data
Main Muscle Worked: Triceps
Other Muscles Worked: None
Equipment: Cable
Mechanics Type: Isolation
   Tips: With your right hand, grasp a stirrup handle attached to the high-cable pulley using an underhand grip. You should be standing directly in front of the weight stack. Pull the handle down so that your upper arm and elbow are locked in to the side of your body and your upper arm and forearm form a right angle. Feeling the contraction in your triceps, pull the stirrup handle down to your side until your arm is straight. Squeeze and then slowly return the handle to the starting position. Finish your desired number of reps, then switch arms.

Cable Incline Triceps Extension
Exercise Data
Main Muscle Worked: Triceps
Other Muscles Worked: None
Equipment: Cable
Mechanics Type: Isolation

Tips: Preparation: Grasp cable bar from behind with a narrow overhand grip. Position your elbows overhead. **Execution:** Extend your forearm overhead. Lower and repeat.

Lying Dumbbell Tricep Extension
Exercise Data
Main Muscle Worked: Triceps
Other Muscles Worked: None
Equipment: Dumbbell
Mechanics Type: Isolation

Tips: Lay down on a flat bench with your head at the very end of the bench. Hold a dumbbell around the end with both hands (palms facing up). Your arms should be pointed almost straight up, but tilted a little towards your head. While keeping your upper arms and elbows completely still, lower the dumbbell until it is behind your head. Do not let your elbows flare outward. Slowly lift the dumbbell back to the starting position where your elbows are locked or nearly locked. Repeat.

Dumbbell One Arm Triceps Extension
Exercise Data
Main Muscle Worked: Triceps
Other Muscles Worked: None
Equipment: Dumbbell
Mechanics Type: Isolation

Tips: Preparation: Position the dumbbell behind your neck with your elbow positioned upward. **Execution:** Extend your arm until straight. Return and repeat. Continue with opposite arm.

Kneeling Cable Concentration Triceps Extension
Exercise Data
Main Muscle Worked: Triceps
99Other Muscles Worked: None
Equipment: Cable
Mechanics Type: Isolation
   Tips: Hold a stirrup handle attachment that is connected to a high pulley with your right hand. Kneel on your left knee with your left side toward the machine. Keep your right knee bent and your upper thigh parallel to the floor. Keep your right elbow and upper arm against your inner thigh at all time. Extend your arm down in a semicircular motion until arm is vertical and your elbow is locked. Return slowly to the starting position.

Hammer Curls
Exercise Data
Main Muscle Worked: Biceps
Other Muscles Worked: Forearms
Equipment: Dumbbell
Mechanics Type: Isolation
   Tips: With a dumbbell in each hand, stand with your arms hanging at your sides, palms facing each other. Keep your elbows locked into your sides. Your upper body and elbows should remain in the same place during the whole lift. Keeping your palms facing each other, curl the weight in your right hand up in a semi-circle toward your right shoulder. Squeeze the biceps hard at the top of the lift and then slowly lower. Do not turn your wrists during this lift! You can also do one arm at a time and/or alternate.

Reverse Barbell Curl
Exercise Data
Main Muscle Worked: Forearms
Other Muscles Worked: Biceps
Equipment: Barbell
Mechanics Type: Isolation
   Tips: Grasp bar with a shoulder width over hand grip. With the elbows to the side, raise the bar until forearms are vertical. Lower until the arms are fully

extended. Repeat. When the elbow is fully flexed, the elbow should only travel forward a few inches allowing the forearm to be no more than perpendicular to the floor to allow for a relative release of tension in the muscles between repetitions.

Seated Close-Grip Concentration Barbell Curl
Exercise Data
Main Muscle Worked: Biceps
Other Muscles Worked: None
Equipment: Barbell
Mechanics Type: Isolation
    Tips: Place barbell on the floor near the end of a bench. Sit at the end of the bench with your feet about 24 inches apart. Bend forward at the waist, hold bar with both hands, palms up, about 6 inches apart. Rest elbows on your inner thighs about 4 inches up from your knees. Curl bar up in a semicircular motion until your forearms touch your biceps. Go down using the same path. Do not move your torso or upper arms during the lift!

Preacher Curl
Exercise Data
Main Muscle Worked: Biceps
Other Muscles Worked: None
Equipment: Barbell
Mechanics Type: Isolation
    Tips: Using a preacher curl bench and an EZ curl bar, make sure the seat is adjusted to the right height. When you sit, the seat should not be so low that the shoulders are elevated nor so high that you're hunched over the pad. Grasp the bar using a shoulder width grip. Curl the bar upward in an arc. As you begin, be careful not to swing or rock to get it moving. The goal is to make the exercise hard on the biceps. Curl the bar towards your chin, but keep in mind that the resistance is greater at the beginning of the rep. Go down SLOWLY and work the muscle on the way down as well. Can also be done with two dumbbells or one arm at a time.

Hack Squat
Exercise Data
Main Muscle Worked: Quadriceps
Other Muscles Worked: Hamstrings, Calves
Equipment: Machine
Mechanics Type: Compound

Tips: Lie face up on a hack squat machine with shoulders against pad. Place feet on platform. Your feet should be together, toes pointed slightly out. Extend hips and knees. Release dock levers. Flex hips and knees to descend until knees are just short of complete flexion. Raise sled by extending knees and hips. Repeat. Great for developing the lower area of the thigh.

Front Barbell Squat To A Bench
Exercise Data
Main Muscle Worked: Quadriceps
Other Muscles Worked: Hamstrings, Calves
Equipment: Barbell
Mechanics Type: Compound

Tips: Same as the normal Front Barbell Squat but you put a flat bench behind you. Squat down and barely touch the bench. Do NOT sit on it or rest at all. It is just there to help make sure you go all the way down on each repetition. Can also be done with your heels on a 2 X 4.

Front Barbell Squat
Exercise Data
Main Muscle Worked: Quadriceps
Other Muscles Worked: Hamstrings, Calves
Equipment: Barbell
Mechanics Type: Compound

Tips: Place a barbell on your upper chest and rest it on your front deltoids and upper thorax. Place right hand on the bar even with your left deltoid and your left hand on the bar even with your right deltoid. Keep your upper arms slightly above parallel to keep the bar from sliding. Keep your head up and your back straight with a shoulder width stance. Your toes and knees should be slightly pointed outwards. Squat down until your upper thighs are parallel to the floor.

Return slowly to the starting position. Can also be done with your heels on a 1 inch block or with a wider stance.

Barbell Full Squat
Exercise Data
Main Muscle Worked: Quadriceps
Other Muscles Worked: Hamstrings, Calves, Glutes
Equipment: Barbell
Mechanics Type: Compound

Tips: Position a barbell on the back of the shoulders and grasp bar to the sides. Put your feet at shoulder width with your toes and knees slightly pointed outwards. Descend until knees and hips are fully bent. Extend knees and hips until legs are straight. Return and repeat. Some people believe this is damaging to your knee, but others believe it is a great exercise. Can also be done with dumbbells in your hands instead or on the Smith machine.

Barbell Squat
Exercise Data
Main Muscle Worked: Quadriceps Other Muscles Worked: Lower Back, Hamstrings, Calves, Glutes Equipment: Barbell Mechanics Type: Compound

Tips: Rest a barbell on the upper portion of your back, not your neck. Firmly grip the bar with your hands almost twice your shoulder width apart. Position your feet about shoulder width apart and your toes should be pointing just a little outward with your knees in the same direction. Keep your back as straight as possible and your chin up, bend your knees and slowly lower your hips straight down until your THIGHS ARE PARALLEL TO THE FLOOR. Once you reach the bottom position, press the weight up back to the starting position. Don't lean over or curve your back forward! You can use a Belt to help reduce the chance of lower back injury. You can put your heels on a 1 inch block to further work the quads. You can also use a wider stance to work the inner quads even more.

Learn More About This Exercise: View Guide

Lying Machine Squat
Exercise Data
Main Muscle Worked: Quadriceps
Other Muscles Worked: Hamstrings, Calves
Equipment: Machine
Mechanics Type: Compound
    Tips: Using a machine like the one shown above, follow the directions that are listed on it.

Narrow Stance Leg Press
Exercise Data
Main Muscle Worked: Quadriceps Other Muscles Worked: Hamstrings, Calves
Equipment: Machine Mechanics Type: Compound
    Tips: Sitting on a leg press machine, position your feet together against the crosspiece about 6 inches apart and toes pointed slightly outward. Grasp the handle grips or sides of the seat. Bend your knees and lower the weight as far as possible without changing the position of your hips. Do not lower the weight so far that your hips start to curl up off the seat! Then slowly push the weight back up using your heels, not your toes. Do not lock your knees at the top, but rather take the weight to just before lock. Then being to lower the weight again SLOWLY. You can change your foot positions to vary the angle on the muscle.

Barbell Seated Calf Raise
Exercise Data
Main Muscle Worked: Calves
Other Muscles Worked: None
Equipment: Barbell
Mechanics Type: Isolation
    Tips: Place a block about 12 inches in front of a flat bench. Sit on the bench and place the balls of your feet on the block. Place a barbell over your upper thighs about 3 inches above your knees. Raise up on your toes as high as possible and squeeze the calves. Lower down to the starting position and stretch as far as you can. Repeat.

Lying Leg Curls
Exercise Data
Main Muscle Worked: Hamstrings
Other Muscles Worked: None
Equipment: Machine
Mechanics Type: Isolation

Tips: Lie face down on a leg-curl machine and hook your heels under the roller pad. Your legs should be stretched out straight so that the pads rest on the back of your ankles. Grasp the handles under the bench for support. Remaining flat on the bench, curl your legs up until your hamstrings are fully contracted. Release and lower the weight slowly back to the starting position. Concentrate on using a full range of motion and do not SWING the weight up. You can point your toes to intensify the burn in your hamstrings.

Cable Hip Adduction
Exercise Data
Main Muscle Worked: Quadriceps
Other Muscles Worked: None
Equipment: Cable
Mechanics Type: Isolation

Tips: Preparation: Stand in front of low pulley facing to one side. Attach the cable cuff to near ankle. Step out away from the stack with a wide stance and grasp ballet bar. Stand on your far foot and allow near leg to be Pulled toward low pulley.

Execution: Move near leg just in front of far leg by abducting your hip. Return and repeat. Turn around and continue with the opposite leg.

Seated Calf Raise
Exercise Data
Main Muscle Worked: Calves
Other Muscles Worked: None
Equipment: Machine
Mechanics Type: Isolation

Tips: Sit on a calf raise machine. Place your upper thighs under the leg pad just above your knees. Disengage any weight lock that may be in place.

Lower your heels to the lowest possible position. Slowly raise up on your toes as high as you can go. Hold for a moment and return to the starting position. Do not "swing" the weight up using momentum! Repeat.

Lateral Raise - With Bands
Exercise Data
Main Muscle Worked: Shoulders
Other Muscles Worked: Triceps, Lats
Equipment: Other
Mechanics Type: Compound
Tips: Stand on band so tension begins with arms at sides. Keeping your arms straight, raise you arms out to your sides so they are parallel with the floor.

Machine Shoulder (Military) Press
Exercise Data
Main Muscle Worked: Shoulders
Other Muscles Worked: Triceps
Equipment: Machine
Mechanics Type: Compound
Tips: Follow the directions on the shoulder press machine.

Barbell Incline Shoulder Raise
Exercise Data
Main Muscle Worked: Shoulders
Other Muscles Worked: Triceps
Equipment: Barbell
Mechanics Type: Compound
Tips:
Preparation: Lie Horizontal on an incline bench. Lift barbell from rack with a shoulder width overhand grip. Position barbell over the upper chest with elbows extended.
Execution: Raises your shoulders toward the bar as high as possible. Lower shoulders to bench and repeat.

Lying One-Arm Lateral Raise
Exercise Data
Main Muscle Worked: Shoulders
Other Muscles Worked: Lats
Equipment: Dumbbell
Mechanics Type: Isolation
Tips: Lie on your side on a flat bench with a dumbbell in your uppermost hand. Your shoulders should be perpendicular to the bench. The lower arm should be extended in a comfortable position to act as a counterbalance. Your upper leg should be straight in line with the bench and your lower leg should stretch out to the floor to stabilize yourself. Start by extending the dumbbell out in front of your body and slightly toward the floor. Using your shoulder muscles, raise the weight directly above your body, then lower to the starting position. Finish your reps and then switch sides. Don't use weights that are too heavy or you will not be isolating the shoulder as much.

Front Two-Dumbbell Raise
Exercise Data
Main Muscle Worked: Shoulders
Other Muscles Worked: None
Equipment: Dumbbell
Mechanics Type: Isolation
Tips: Same as the Front Dumbbell Raise but with both arms at the same time. Can also be done with a barbell.

Front Dumbbell Raise
Exercise Data
Main Muscle Worked: Shoulders
Other Muscles Worked: None
Equipment: Dumbbell
Mechanics Type: Isolation
Tips: Stand with a dumbbell in each hand, palms facing backward. Your feet should be about shoulder width apart. Maintain a slight bend in your elbows throughout the exercise so that your arms are straight, but not quite locked. Lift the weight in your left hand in front of you in a wide arc until it is slightly higher

than shoulder height. With a smooth, controlled motion, lower the weight while simultaneously lifting the weight in your right hand, so that both arms are in motion at the same time. Do not cheat by swinging or leaning backwards! Can also be done with two dumbbells at the same time or a barbell.

Front Cable Raise
Exercise Data
Main Muscle Worked: Shoulders
Other Muscles Worked: None
Equipment: Cable
Mechanics Type: Isolation
Tips: Works the front delts. Grasp the cable attachment that is attached to the low pulley with one hand. Face away from the pulley and put your arm straight down. Keeping your body straight and your elbow nearly locked, raise your arm up in front of your body. Do not swing! Go up to about eye level, then slowly return to the starting position. Finish your reps and then switch arms.

Donkey Calf Raises
Exercise Data
Main Muscle Worked: Calves
Other Muscles Worked: None
Equipment: Other
Mechanics Type: Isolation
Tips: Many of you may have seen Arnold do this in his hayday, but how many of you actually know that it was called Donkey calf raises or even do them? I'll just give you a quick run through on how to perform them. First, go to a gym with obese people. (lol, alright, I'm joking, but they do accelerate calf development while doing this exercise!) Ok, lean over on a knee height or slightly lower bench/platform, forming an 'L' shape with your torso and lower body. Have a calf raise platform or a thick Olympic weight at the bottom of your feet, tip-toeing on them. Get a few buddies to sit on your back, like they do when horse riding and start repping out some donkey calf raises!

Dips - Chest Version
Exercise Data
Main Muscle Worked: Chest
Other Muscles Worked: Triceps, Shoulders
Equipment: Body Only
Mechanics Type: Compound
Tips: Same as the Triceps Version, except you are leaning forward, which works more of the lower chest. Using the parallel bars, grip the handles and push yourself up to your starting position. With elbows close to body and hips straight, lower body until shoulders are slightly stretched. Push body up in same posture and repeat. You can bend and cross your legs or keep them straight. You can add weight by using a Dip Belt.

Calf Press On The Leg Press Machine
Exercise Data
Main Muscle Worked: Calves
Other Muscles Worked: None
Equipment: Machine
Mechanics Type: Isolation
Tips: While sitting a leg press machine, press the weight rack up as if you were going to do a leg press. Lock your knees and slide your feet down so that only the balls of your feet are on the rack and your heels are hanging off. Push with your toes and point the feet like a ballet stance, pushing the rack along with you. Let the rack come back down bringing the toes closer to your body and repeat. Make sure the handles remain in the locked position. If your feet were to slip off the rack and you don't have the handles locked you can be injured. Don't bounce the rack up and down. Use the muscles slowly with control. You can also focus on the inner or outer calves by pointing your toes in or out instead of keeping them straight.

Calf Raises - With Bands
Exercise Data
Main Muscle Worked: Calves
Other Muscles Worked: None

Equipment: Other
Mechanics Type: Isolation
Tips: Stand on a band so that the tension begins with hands by shoulders and standing straight up. (Make sure you are standing on the band with your toes). Keeping hands by your shoulder, stand up on your toes as you would with a barbell calf raise.

DAILY JOURNAL/ BIBILE STUDY

One of the hardest things that I had to come to realize was the benefit of documenting my journey through this war. The value of a daily journal was lost to me until I started working on this program. It was during this process that I began to write more than just my workout notes or my meals. I started documenting my emotional struggles and my spiritual notes.

This is when I understood the purpose of this journal. How could I keep track of my growth, both spiritually and emotionally? The best way was to keep a daily journal of my journey.

Therefore I strongly feel that you, dear warrior, will find the same value in keeping a daily journal of your battle. I have included in this chapter some help for those of you who are struggling with this part of the program.

When you start working on this journal I want to suggest that you put in a picture of yourself at the starting point of your diet. Keep this in the front of the journal. Write on the back where your weight is, what size clothes your wearing, and how you are emotionally. You may want to add your spiritual assessment.

Remember to be honest with yourself. This is not the time to hide your feelings. Now the goal is to maintain a daily journal. Daily, is the key word here.

Start each day with your notes on how you feel emotionally. Document your first meal. Put down your goals and the times for your workout.

When you finish the day write down your emotional feelings. Then be honest about if you were able to stay on the diet. Did you do your full workout? If not, why did you stop short? All of these things will help you on your journey through this battle.

So the next few pages will have some format suggestions for your journal. I have included some questions to help you get started. I have also included a devotional guide to help with your spiritual food. You will find this in the second half of this chapter. I have set this up for a twelve month guide through the Bible. I would suggest that you check out some of the local book stores for some additional help with both a devotional guide and some Journals. I hope that this will give you a starting point.

DEAR DIARY:

Today I woke up and the first thing on my mind was......

I have planned to work out at.....

My goal today is to......

Breakfast....

Lunch.....

Dinner.....

I read in scripture.....

I feel that God is saying.....

It's time for bed and I really battled with.....

I finished my workout but I wasn't able to do.....

I feel like.....

Now in this guide I hope you can see how honesty is vitally important when writing this journal. I will add that honesty should be easier when you know that this is strictly for your own viewing. It is not to be shared with others unless you feel it necessary.

There may be times when this is needed for your own growth. I would suggest that it be limited to people that you know would not violate your privacy. Be sure that the items that you reveal within your journal are things that you are prompted to write by the guidance of the Holy Spirit.

Bible Study

Focus is the hardest part of dieting. We are so used to focusing on ourselves that we find it hard to focus on God. But this is the best time to turn our focus away from our own wants and put them back on our Creator.

I have struggled trying to find a good Bible study guide to help develop the right devotional for you. It has been a search of trial and error. Much of the error being my own. But I have finally gathered the right information to help you with your devotional time.

Understand, as I have said through this whole book, I am only giving you a suggestion. Do not consider this the only appropriate Bible study. If you have already begun a daily devotional or know of one that you would feel more comfortable using please do.

I have laid out this study to incorporate both the Old and New Testaments and I will be using the King James Version, the New American Standard and the Amplified. I am doing this because I want you to get the full meaning of the scripture reference.

Some of the quotes I will be using will be from friends, family, and from pastors who have been an influence in my life. Please take this into consideration. These people have had a great impact on my life and I consider them crucial to my becoming the man that I am today.

As I have begun developing this whole daily devotional I have felt the Lord leading me to an anagram that speaks the message of the Reality Weight Loss philosophy. That word is *R.E.S.T.O.R.E.*

You see, I believe that God is a God of *restoration.* He can and will restore us spiritually, emotionally, and physically to the people that He desires us to become.

So if we understand that and believe that we need to take this step ;and begin to put the word *restore* into daily practice; we need to ask how can we do this? Well, follow with me through this daily devotional that will teach us how to live out *restoration.*

SUNDAY   RECOGNIZE OUR SIN:

Psalm 51:1-14 New King James Version (NKJV)

A Prayer of Repentance

To the Chief Musician. A Psalm of David when Nathan the prophet went to him, after he had gone in to Bathsheba.

51Have mercy upon me, O God, According to Your lovingkindness; According to the multitude of Your tender mercies, Blot out my transgressions.

2 Wash me thoroughly from my iniquity, And cleanse me from my sin.

3 For I acknowledge my transgressions, And my sin is always before me.

4 Against You, You only, have I sinned, And done this evil in Your sight— That You may be found just when You speak,[a]And blameless when You judge.

5 Behold, I was brought forth in iniquity, And in sin my mother conceived me.

6 Behold, You desire truth in the inward parts, And in the hidden part You will make me to know wisdom. Purge me with hyssop, and I shall be clean; Wash me, and I shall be whiter than snow.

8 Make me hear joy and gladness, That the bones You have broken may rejoice.

9 Hide Your face from my sins, And blot out all my iniquities.

10 Create in me a clean heart, O God, And renew a steadfast spirit within me.

11 Do not cast me away from Your presence, And do not take Your Holy Spirit from me.

12 Restore to me the joy of Your salvation, And uphold me by Your generous Spirit.

13 Then I will teach transgressors Your ways, And sinners shall be converted to You.

14 Deliver me from the guilt of bloodshed, O God, The God of my salvation, And my tongue shall sing aloud of Your righteousness.

Psalm 51:1-14 Amplified Bible (AMP)

Psalm 51

To the Chief Musician. A Psalm of David; when Nathan the prophet came to him after he had sinned with Bathsheba.

1 Have mercy upon me, O God, according to Your steadfast love; according to the multitude of Your tender mercy and loving-kindness blot out my transgressions.

2 Wash me thoroughly [and repeatedly] from my iniquity and guilt and cleanse me and make me wholly pure from my sin!

3 For I am conscious of my transgressions and I acknowledge them; my sin is ever before me.

4 Against You, You only, have I sinned and done that which is evil in Your sight, so that You are justified in Your sentence and faultless in Your judgment.

5 Behold, I was brought forth in [a state of] iniquity; my mother was sinful who conceived me [and I too am sinful].

6 Behold, You desire truth in the inner being; make me therefore to know wisdom in my inmost heart.

7 Purify me with hyssop, and I shall be clean [ceremonially]; wash me, and I shall [in reality] be whiter than snow.

8 Make me to hear joy and gladness and be satisfied; let the bones which You have broken rejoice.

9 Hide Your face from my sins and blot out all my guilt and iniquities.

10 Create in me a clean heart, O God, and renew a right, persevering, and steadfast spirit within me.

11 Cast me not away from Your presence and take not Your Holy Spirit from me.

12 Restore to me the joy of Your salvation and uphold me with a willing spirit.

13 Then will I teach transgressors Your ways, and sinners shall be converted and return to You.

14 Deliver me from bloodguiltiness and death, O God, the God of my salvation, and my tongue shall sing aloud of Your righteousness (Your rightness and Your justice).

The hardest part of our battle, as obese people, is recognizing the truth of our sin. Remember that this was our first revelation in this book. Obesity, is rooted in rebellion. Whether it is rebellion to our bodies, our past, or our present. We need to confess this before the Father and allow Him to **restore** us unto Himself.

"**For I acknowledge my transgressions: and my sin is ever before me.**" David confronts the truth of his sin and confesses it before God. He understands that his sin was directly related to his walk with God.

Read the story of David and Bathsheba and you will see how this one sin resulted in the literal collapse of David's kingdom. This was a man who had been called the **"friend of God"**. He was chosen by God to lead the people of Israel. He battled hundreds and overcame the great Goliath. He saw the power of God on a daily basis, yet one sin brought him to his knees.

Nathan spoke the word of God to David.

1 Samuel 12:7-14 New King James Version (NKJV)

7 Now therefore, stand still, that I may reason with you before the LORD concerning all the righteous acts of the LORD which He did to you and your fathers:

8 When Jacob had gone into Egypt,[a] and your fathers cried out to the LORD, then the LORD sent Moses and Aaron, who brought your fathers out of Egypt and made them dwell in this place.

9 And when they forgot the LORD their God, He sold them into the hand of Sisera, commander of the army of Hazor, into the hand of the Philistines, and into the hand of the king of Moab; and they fought against them.

10 Then they cried out to the LORD, and said, 'We have sinned, because we have forsaken the LORD and served the Baals and Ashtoreths;[b]but now deliver us from the hand of our enemies, and we will serve You.'

11 And the LORD sent Jerubbaal,[c] Bedan,[d] Jephthah, and Samuel,[e] and delivered you out of the hand of your enemies on every side; and you dwelt in safety.

12 And when you saw that Nahash king of the Ammonites came against you, you said to me, 'No, but a king shall reign over us,' when the LORD your God was your king.

13 "Now therefore, here is the king whom you have chosen and whom you have desired. And take note, the LORD has set a king over you.

14 If you fear the LORD and serve Him and obey His voice, and do not rebel against the commandment of the LORD, then both you and the king who reigns over you will continue following the LORD your God.

1 Samuel 12:7-14 Amplified Bible (AMP)

7 Now present yourselves, that I may plead with you before the Lord concerning all the righteous acts of the Lord which He did for you and for your fathers.

8 When Jacob and his sons had come into Egypt [and the Egyptians oppressed them], and your fathers cried to the Lord, then the Lord sent Moses and Aaron, who brought forth your fathers out of Egypt and made them dwell in this place.

9 But when they forgot the Lord their God, He sold them into the hand of Sisera, commander of Hazor's army, and into the hands of the Philistines and of the king of Moab, and they fought those foes.

10 And they cried to the Lord, saying, We have sinned because we have forsaken the Lord and have served the Baals and the Ashtaroth; but now deliver us from the hands of our enemies, and we will serve You.

11 And the Lord sent Jerubbaal and Barak and Jephthah and Samuel, and He delivered you out of the hands of your enemies on every side, and you dwelt safely.

12 But when you saw that Nahash king of the Ammonites came against you, you said to me, No! A king shall reign over us—when the Lord your God was your King!

13 Now see the king whom you have chosen and for whom you have asked; behold, the Lord has set a king over you.

14 If you will revere and fear the Lord and serve Him and hearken to His voice and not rebel against His commandment, and if both you and your king will follow the Lord your God, it will be good!

When David was suddenly confronted with the sin in his life he fell on his face. The sin that he had committed could have been swept under the rug. Being real, we know that David could have simply eliminated the truth and gone on his way. But the realization of just how this sin had effected his walk with God was overwhelming.

We are in a constant struggle with the truth in our lives. Whether we are battling obesity or battling some other hidden sin. We try and hide every part of that sin and yet it is obvious to those around us just how it is effecting our relationship with others and more importantly, with God.

In this study, I ask you to recognize where you are with God. Look at the mirror dear reader. Confess the sin that has brought you to this place. Accept the healing that God desires to do in your life.

I find myself confronted with the truth of my walk. This is my life. I was a David. I loved the Lord and served Him with everything in me. Yet my sin was clear to those around me. My brothers and sisters in Christ tried to confront me with my sin and I ignored them. So God had to bring me to a place where I was broken and able to listen to the Holy Spirit.

There He has begun to initiate a healing in my spirit and my emotion. Now I have found that the Lord is also going further and healing me physically. Although the damage done to my body through my obesity has been extensive I have found that my high blood pressure is slowly improving and my diabetes is beginning to come under control.

I want to leave you today with the truth that God is faithful in His promises. He has promised to never leave us or forsake us. He has promised to hold us in

His hand and that nothing can take us out of His hand. This means that nothing or no one even ourselves. So rejoice in this truth. Take today and just praise God for His faithfulness. Know that no matter what you have done or what has been done to you, You are God's.

Psalm 51:1-12 New King James Version (NKJV)
A Prayer of Repentance
To the Chief Musician. A Psalm of David when Nathan the prophet went to him, after he had gone in to Bathsheba.

51 Have mercy upon me, O God, According to Your lovingkindness; According to the multitude of Your tender mercies, Blot out my transgressions.

2 Wash me thoroughly from my iniquity, And cleanse me from my sin.

3 For I acknowledge my transgressions, And my sin is always before me.

4 Against You, You only, have I sinned, And done this evil in Your sight— That You may be found just when You speak,[a] And blameless when You judge.

5 Behold, I was brought forth in iniquity, And in sin my mother conceived me.

6 Behold, You desire truth in the inward parts, And in the hidden part You will make me to know wisdom.

7 Purge me with hyssop, and I shall be clean; Wash me, and I shall be whiter than snow.

8 Make me hear joy and gladness, That the bones You have broken may rejoice.

9 Hide Your face from my sins, And blot out all my iniquities.

10 Create in me a clean heart, O God, And renew a steadfast spirit within me.

11 Do not cast me away from Your presence, And do not take Your Holy Spirit from me.

12 Restore to me the joy of Your salvation, And uphold me by Your generous Spirit.

Psalm 51:1-12 Amplified Bible (AMP)
Psalm 51

To the Chief Musician. A Psalm of David; when Nathan the prophet came to him after he had sinned with Bathsheba.

1 Have mercy upon me, O God, according to Your steadfast love; according to the multitude of Your tender mercy and loving-kindness blot out my transgressions.

2 Wash me thoroughly [and repeatedly] from my iniquity and guilt and cleanse me and make me wholly pure from my sin!

3 For I am conscious of my transgressions and I acknowledge them; my sin is ever before me.

4 Against You, You only, have I sinned and done that which is evil in Your sight, so that You are justified in Your sentence and faultless in Your judgment.

5 Behold, I was brought forth in [a state of] iniquity; my mother was sinful who conceived me [and I too am sinful].

6 Behold, You desire truth in the inner being; make me therefore to know wisdom in my inmost heart.

7 Purify me with hyssop, and I shall be clean [ceremonially]; wash me, and I shall [in reality] be whiter than snow.

8 Make me to hear joy and gladness and be satisfied; let the bones which You have broken rejoice.

9 Hide Your face from my sins and blot out all my guilt and iniquities.

10 Create in me a clean heart, O God, and renew a right, persevering, and steadfast spirit within me.

11 Cast me not away from Your presence and take not Your Holy Spirit from me.

12 Restore to me the joy of Your salvation and uphold me with a willing spirit.

Take the following lines and write down your thoughts on the passage.

MONDAY   EVALUATE OUR WALK WITH GOD:

What does it mean to evaluate? What this means is that you place a model next to yourself and compare to see what is lacking. But what model do we use?

1 Corinthians 3:7-15 New King James Version (NKJV)

7 So then neither he who plants is anything, nor he who waters, but God who gives the increase.

8 Now he who plants and he who waters are one, and each one will receive his own reward according to his own labor.

9 For we are God's fellow workers; you are God's field, you are God's building.

10 According to the grace of God which was given to me, as a wise master builder I have laid the foundation, and another builds on it. But let each one take heed how he builds on it.

11 For no other foundation can anyone lay than that which is laid, which is Jesus Christ.

12 Now if anyone builds on this foundation with gold, silver, precious stones, wood, hay, straw,

13 each one's work will become clear; for the Day will declare it, because it will be revealed by fire; and the fire will test each one's work, of what sort it is.

14 If anyone's work which he has built on it endures, he will receive a reward.

15 If anyone's work is burned, he will suffer loss; but he himself will be saved, yet so as through fire.

1 Corinthians 3:7-15 Amplified Bible (AMP)

7 So neither he who plants is anything nor he who waters, but [only] God Who makes it grow andbecome greater.

8 He who plants and he who waters are equal (one in aim, of the same importance and esteem), yet each shall receive his own reward (wages), according to his own labor.

9 For we are fellow workmen (joint promoters, laborers together) with and for God; you are God's[a]garden and vineyard and field under cultivation, [you are] God's building.

10 According to the grace (the special endowment for my task) of God bestowed on me, like a skillful architect and master builder I laid [the] foundation, and now another [man] is building upon it. But let each [man] be careful how he builds upon it,

11 For no other foundation can anyone lay than that which is [already] laid, which is Jesus Christ (the Messiah, the Anointed One).

12 But if anyone builds upon the Foundation, whether it be with gold, silver, precious stones, wood, hay, straw,

13 The work of each [one] will become [plainly, openly] known (shown for what it is); for the day [of Christ] will disclose and declare it, because it will be revealed with fire, and the fire will test andcritically appraise the character and worth of the work each person has done.

14 If the work which any person has built on this Foundation [any product of his efforts whatever] survives [this test], he will get his reward.

15 But if any person's work is burned up [under the test], he will suffer the loss [of it all, losing his reward], though he himself will be saved, but only as [one who has passed] through fire.

In my youth I would often build model cars. I have always had a fascination with hot rods, and this was my way of owning the cars that I could not afford. When building these cars I would take out an instruction guide that would show me where each piece was meant to go.

Often these pieces were very small and hard to identify. The only way that I could be sure I had the right piece was to compare it with the picture in the instructions.

In our daily life we are confronted with choices that need to be made. As we diet, we must choose the right foods. As we work we must choose to be honest, or not. In each decision, we have a model to base that choice upon.

Our model is the life of Jesus Christ. In the book of John, Jesus is quoted saying in 5:19, " Then answered Jesus and said unto them, ' Verily, verily, I say unto you, The Son can do nothing of Himself, but what He seeth the Father do: for what things soever He doeth, these also doeth the Son likewise."

Clearly we see that even Christ Himself examined His actions to be sure that He was moving only as the Father directed. He compared His actions to those of His Father.

So I leave you with this thought for today. If you are comparing your daily walk to that of the life of Christ, how does is match up? Now write your thoughts about he previous verses.

TUESDAY   SATURATE OUR LIVES WITH PRAISE:

I will admit that this is a subject that it is hard for me not to get upon a soapbox over. I am a worshiper. I lead worship at my church and have been involved in some form of praise and worship in church for most of my life.

The main point is that I have seen just how powerful true worship can be in the life of the believer. We have forgotten that God calls for His people to praise Him daily. What I want you to understand is just how precious your praise is to God.

Read in the following passage the words of the prophet Joel as he talks about praise.

Joel 2:23-32 New King James Version (NKJV)
23 Be glad then, you children of Zion,And rejoice in the LORD your God; For He has given you the former rain faithfully,[a] And He will cause the rain to come down for you—The former rain,
And the latter rain in the first month.
24 The threshing floors shall be full of wheat, And the vats shall overflow with new wine and oil.
25 "So I will restore to you the years that the swarming locust has eaten, The crawling locust,
The consuming locust, And the chewing locust,[b] My great army which I sent among you.
26 You shall eat in plenty and be satisfied, And praise the name of the LORD your God, Who has dealt wondrously with you; And My people shall never be put to shame.
27 Then you shall know that I am in the midst of Israel: I am the LORD your God And there is no other. My people shall never be put to shame.
    God's Spirit Poured Out
28 "And it shall come to pass afterward That I will pour out My Spirit on all flesh; Your sons and your daughters shall prophesy, Your old men shall dream dreams, Your young men shall see visions.

29 And also on My menservants and on My maidservants I will pour out My Spirit in those days.

30 "And I will show wonders in the heavens and in the earth: Blood and fire and pillars of smoke.

31 The sun shall be turned into darkness, And the moon into blood, Before the coming of the great and awesome day of the LORD.

32 And it shall come to pass That whoever calls on the name of the LORD Shall be saved.
For in Mount Zion and in Jerusalem there shall be deliverance, As the LORD has said, Among the remnant whom the LORD calls.
Joel 2:23-32 Amplified Bible (AMP)

23 Be glad then, you children of Zion, and rejoice in the Lord, your God; for He gives you the former orearly rain in just measure and in righteousness, and He causes to come down for you the rain, the former rain and the latter rain, as before.

24 And the [threshing] floors shall be full of grain and the vats shall overflow with juice [of the grape] and oil.

25 And I will restore or replace for you the years that the locust has eaten —the hopping locust, the stripping locust, and the crawling locust, My great army which I sent among you.

26 And you shall eat in plenty and be satisfied and praise the name of the Lord, your God, Who has dealt wondrously with you. And My people shall never be put to shame.

27 And you shall know, understand, and realize that I am in the midst of Israel and that I the Lord am your God and there is none else. My people shall never be put to shame.

28 And afterward I will pour out My Spirit upon all flesh; and your sons and your daughters shall prophesy, your old men shall dream dreams, your young men shall see visions.

29 Even upon the menservants and upon the maidservants in those days will I pour out My Spirit.

30 And I will show signs and wonders in the heavens, and on the earth, blood and fire and columns of smoke.

31 The sun shall be turned to darkness and the moon to blood before the great and terrible day of the Lord comes.

32 And whoever shall call on the name of the Lord shall be delivered and saved, for in Mount Zion and in Jerusalem there shall be those who escape, as the Lord has said, and among the remnant [of survivors] shall be those whom the Lord calls.

This is one of the favorite passages for many of today's preachers. But I think that the message is also very exciting for the average Christian to catch. Just look at this dear friend and read how God is pouring upon you His Spirit.

Consider this dear believer. Know that God has blessed you with His Spirit to empower you on a daily basis.

Do you come upon times that everything is just too overwhelming for you?

Do you ever feel like you just can't make it through?

Are you facing a day when the temptations have just come from every side and you don't feel like you can make it another day?

Don't be afraid dear brother or sister. Rejoice for God has given you His Spirit. He says that all those things that the enemy has stolen from you, He will return them to you. He has said that He will not allow you to ever be ashamed.

How does this effect your life today?

_____
_____
_____
_____
_____
_____
_____
_____
_____
_____
_____
_____

WEDNESDAY   TEAR DOWN THE STRONGHOLD:

Tearing down the strongholds in our lives is one of the hardest things that the Holy Spirit asks us to do. This has been something that I have battled over for many years. One of the hardest parts of my own process has been confronting those areas that God desires broken.

Strongholds take many forms. Some of them have been put in our hearts by others. Some of them by our own decisions. Either way they have taken up residence in our lives and control our decision making process. Let's look at this story in the book of Nehemiah.

In this time Nehemiah had left Jerusalem in the hands of Eliashib. Nehemiah had returned to Babylon for a short time and trusted Eliashib to take care of the temple. However, upon his return he found that Eliashib had built a small chamber within the temple for Tobiah.

Nehemiah 13:7-11 New King James Version (NKJV)
7 and I came to Jerusalem and discovered the evil that Eliashib had done for Tobiah, in preparing a room for him in the courts of the house of God.
8 And it grieved me bitterly; therefore I threw all the household goods of Tobiah out of the room.
9 Then I commanded them to cleanse the rooms; and I brought back into them the articles of the house of God, with the grain offering and the frankincense.
10 I also realized that the portions for the Levites had not been given them; for each of the Levites and the singers who did the work had gone back to his field.
11 So I contended with the rulers, and said, "Why is the house of God forsaken?" And I gathered them together and set them in their place

Nehemiah 13:7-11 Amplified Bible (AMP)

7 And came to Jerusalem. Then I discovered the evil that Eliashib had done for Tobiah in preparing him [an adversary] a chamber in the courts of the house of God!

8 And it grieved me exceedingly, and I threw all the house furnishings of Tobiah out of the chamber.

9 Then I commanded, and they cleansed the chambers; and I brought back there the vessels of the house of God, with the cereal offerings and the frankincense.

10 And I perceived that the portions of the Levites had not been given them, so that the Levites and the singers who did the work [forced by necessity] had each fled to his field.

11 Then I contended with the officials and said, Why is the house of God neglected *and* forsaken? I gathered the Levites and singers and set them in their stations.

Here we have this priest Eliashib thinking that there is nothing wrong with allowing his buddy Tobiah to set up his apartment in the temple. Now, I am sorry to be blunt but that is just a 'no brainer'. Would you allow a known drug dealer or local drunk to have himself an apartment right in the middle of the local church? Of course not!

But putting this into the perspective of our hearts and daily spiritual walk, we do the same thing. Paul explains that the church in Corinth had been allowing sin in the church. He tells them that this is a shame not only for them but to God Himself.

1 Corinthians 6:19-20 New King James Version (NKJV)

19 Or do you not know that your body is the temple of the Holy Spirit *who is* in you, whom you have from God, and you are not your own?

20 For you were bought at a price; therefore glorify God in your body[a] and in your spirit, which are God's.

1 Corinthians 6:19-20 Amplified Bible (AMP)

19 Do you not know that your body is the temple (the very sanctuary) of the Holy Spirit Who lives within you, Whom you have received [as a Gift] from God? You are not your own,

20 You were bought with a price [purchased with a [a]preciousness and paid for, [b]made His own]. So then, honor God *and* bring glory to Him in your body.

Paul was telling them that they need to remember they are a living temple. We are also that temple. Yet we have now seen that we allowed Tobiah to set up home within that temple.

Tobiah for us may be unforgiveness, resentment, immorality, or whatever sin that has us under it's control. We have this sin within our walls and it is time to bring down this invader.

What is your personal Tobiah? Can you identify him? Do you need someone to pray through this stronghold with you? Write down your personal thoughts and read them over. Read the whole chapter 6 in 1 Corinthians.

THURSDAY   OPEN OUR HEARTS TO HIS HEALING:

The hardest part of healing is forgiving ourselves. We seem to relish in beating ourselves up on a daily basis. But we need to understand that we are forgiven. For God to do the healing that He desires to do in our lives we must be willing to let Him have free reign

We need to open our hearts up to Him and let Him move through our past and bring those things up to the surface that may be painful but are crucial to our healing. The key point is to allow Him freedom. This is a matter of trusting God completely.

Do you trust God completely?

Paul wrote a letter to the church in Ephesus and spoke of the great love that God had for them. He told them that it was that same love that compelled him to be willing to go to prison for their sake. It is because of this great love that he prays for them everyday.

Ephesians 3:7-19 New King James Version (NKJV)
7 of which I became a minister according to the gift of the grace of God given to me by the effective working of His power.
Purpose of the Mystery
8 To me, who am less than the least of all the saints, this grace was given, that I should preach among the Gentiles the unsearchable riches of Christ,
9 and to make all see what is the fellowship[a]of the mystery, which from the beginning of the ages has been hidden in God who created all things through Jesus Christ;[b]
10 to the intent that now the manifold wisdom of God might be made known by the church to the principalities and powers in the heavenly places,
11 according to the eternal purpose which He accomplished in Christ Jesus our Lord,

12 in whom we have boldness and access with confidence through faith in Him.

13 Therefore I ask that you do not lose heart at my tribulations for you, which is your glory.

Appreciation of the Mystery

14 For this reason I bow my knees to the Father of our Lord Jesus Christ,

[c]

15 from whom the whole family in heaven and earth is named,

16 that He would grant you, according to the riches of His glory, to be strengthened with might through His Spirit in the inner man,

17 that Christ may dwell in your hearts through faith; that you, being rooted and grounded in love,

18 may be able to comprehend with all the saints what is the width and length and depth and height—

19 to know the love of Christ which passes knowledge; that you may be filled with all the fullness of God.

Ephesians 3:7-19 Amplified Bible (AMP)

7 Of this [Gospel] I was made a minister according to the gift of God's free grace (undeserved favor) which was bestowed on me by the exercise (the working in all its effectiveness) of His power.

8 To me, though I am the very least of all the saints (God's consecrated people), this grace (favor, privilege) was granted and graciously entrusted: to proclaim to the Gentiles the unending (boundless, fathomless, incalculable, and exhaustless) riches of Christ [wealth which no human being could have searched out],

9 Also to enlighten all men and make plain to them what is the plan [regarding the Gentiles and providing for the salvation of all men] of the mystery kept hidden through the ages and concealed until now in [the mind of] God Who created all things by Christ Jesus.

10 [The purpose is] that through the church the [a]complicated, many-sided wisdom of God in all its infinite variety and innumerable aspects might now be made known to the angelic rulers and authorities (principalities and powers) in the heavenly sphere.

11 This is in accordance with the terms of the eternal and timeless purpose which He has realized and carried into effect in [the person of] Christ Jesus our Lord,

12 In Whom, because of our faith in Him, we dare to have the boldness (courage and confidence) of free access (an unreserved approach to God with freedom and without fear).

13 So I ask you not to lose heart [not to faint or become despondent through fear] at what I am suffering in your behalf. [Rather glory in it] for it is an honor to you.

14 For this reason [[b]seeing the greatness of this plan by which you are built together in Christ], I bow my knees before the Father of our Lord Jesus Christ,

15 For Whom every family in heaven and on earth is named [that Father from Whom all fatherhood takes its title and derives its name].

16 May He grant you out of the rich treasury of His glory to be strengthened and reinforced with mighty power in the inner man by the [Holy] Spirit [Himself indwelling your innermost being and personality].

17 May Christ through your faith [actually] dwell (settle down, abide, make His permanent home) in your hearts! May you be rooted deep in love and founded securely on love,

18 That you may have the power and be strong to apprehend and grasp with all the saints [God's devoted people, the experience of that love] what is the breadth and length and height and depth [of it];

19 [That you may really come] to know [practically, [c]through experience for yourselves] the love of Christ, which far surpasses [d]mere knowledge [without experience]; that you may be filled [through all your being] [e]unto all the fullness of God [may have the richest measure of the divine Presence, and [f]become a body wholly filled and flooded with God Himself]!

We spend so much time condemning ourselves that we build a wall between us and God. We come to Him with sin that has already been forgiven and covered with the blood of Christ.

Read chapter 8 of the book of Romans and you will see how Paul tells the Roman church that they are not under the condemnation of the law. We also battle with this condemnation. We put ourselves under the law of self. But read this passage from Romans 8.

Romans 8:1-7 New King James Version (NKJV)
Free from Indwelling Sin

8 1There is therefore now no condemnation to those who are in Christ Jesus,[a] who do not walk according to the flesh, but according to the Spirit.

2 For the law of the Spirit of life in Christ Jesus has made me free from the law of sin and death.

3 For what the law could not do in that it was weak through the flesh, God did by sending His own Son in the likeness of sinful flesh, on account of sin: He condemned sin in the flesh,

4 that the righteous requirement of the law might be fulfilled in us who do not walk according to the flesh but according to the Spirit.

5 For those who live according to the flesh set their minds on the things of the flesh, but those who live according to the Spirit, the things of the Spirit.

6 For to be carnally minded is death, but to be spiritually minded is life and peace.

7 Because the carnal mind is enmity against God; for it is not subject to the law of God, nor indeed can be.

Romans 8:37-39 New King James Version (NKJV)

37 Yet in all these things we are more than conquerors through Him who loved us.

38 For I am persuaded that neither death nor life, nor angels nor principalities nor powers, nor things present nor things to come,

39 nor height nor depth, nor any other created thing, shall be able to separate us from the love of God which is in Christ Jesus our Lord.

Romans 8:1-7 Amplified Bible (AMP)

8 Therefore, [there is] now no condemnation (no adjudging guilty of wrong) for those who are in Christ Jesus, who live [and] walk not after the dictates of the flesh, but after the dictates of the Spirit.

2 For the law of the Spirit of life [which is] in Christ Jesus [the law of our new being] has freed me from the law of sin and of death.

3 For God has done what the Law could not do, [its power] being weakened by the flesh [[a]the entire nature of man without the Holy Spirit].

Sending His own Son in the guise of sinful flesh and as an offering for sin, [God] condemned sin in the flesh [[b]subdued, overcame, [c]deprived it of its power over all who accept that sacrifice],

4 So that the righteous and just requirement of the Law might be fully met in us who live and move not in the ways of the flesh but in the ways of the Spirit [our lives governed not by the standards and according to the dictates of the flesh, but controlled by the Holy Spirit].

5 For those who are according to the flesh and are controlled by its unholy desires set their minds onand [d]pursue those things which gratify the flesh, but those who are according to the Spirit and are controlled by the desires of the Spirit set their minds on and [e]seek those things which gratify the [Holy] Spirit.

6 Now the mind of the flesh [which is sense and reason without the Holy Spirit] is death [death that[f]comprises all the miseries arising from sin, both here and hereafter]. But the mind of the [Holy] Spirit is life and [soul] peace [both now and forever].

7 [That is] because the mind of the flesh [with its carnal thoughts and purposes] is hostile to God, for it does not submit itself to God's Law; indeed it cannot.

Romans 8:37-39 Amplified Bible (AMP)

37 Yet amid all these things we are more than conquerors [a]and gain a surpassing victory through Him Who loved us.

38 For I am persuaded beyond doubt (am sure) that neither death nor life, nor angels nor principalities, nor things [b]impending and threatening nor things to come, nor powers,

39 Nor height nor depth, nor anything else in all creation will be able to separate us from the love of God which is in Christ Jesus our Lord.

Paul clearly understands the battle that these believers were going through. If you read in the previous chapter you will see how Paul speaks of his own struggle with the flesh but he clearly glorifies the Lord that he is not dependent on his own flesh for his walk with God.

Do you battle with these things?

Do you understand that God has healed you?

Are you willing to let God move within your life, past and present, to see Him bring healing?

Take the next page and write down your own feelings about these passages.

Read through Romans 7 and 8.

_____
_____
_____
_____
_____
_____
_____
_____
_____
_____
_____
_____
_____
_____
_____
_____
_____
_____
_____
_____
_____
_____
_____
_____
_____
_____
_____

FRIDAY REJOICE IN OUR DELIVERANCE:

We have touched on the power of praise in a previous study. But here we are again.

Praise is true power in the believers life.

Reading through the entire book of Psalms you can see how often praise is mentioned. Understand that often the people of Israel walked into battle with the praisers leading the way.

Praise was crucial to the life of David. It influenced even his time as King of Israel. Read in I Chronicles 13 and you will see the story of when David returned the Arch of the Covenant to Israel.

1 Chronicles 13:8 New King James Version (NKJV)
8 Then David and all Israel played music before God with all their might, with singing, on harps, on stringed instruments, on tambourines, on cymbals, and with trumpets.
1 Chronicles 13:8 Amplified Bible (AMP)
8 And David and all Israel merrily celebrated before God with all their might, with songs and lyres and harps and tambourines and cymbals and trumpets.

David and the people were not ashamed of their behavior. They wanted to proclaim unto all that watched that God was God and He was worthy of praise.

The key for this study is to lead us to praise God specifically for the freedom and deliverance that we have been given. In our praise we can share the gospel and the freedom available through prayer.

Another part of praising God for our deliverance is to remind us of our freedom. So often we battle with the understanding of our freedom that we fall back into our bondage.

We forget that we have been forgiven. We find the enemy creeping around our feet trying to pull us back into the old life. But we have been set free. Is this not true?

Therefore I ask that you focus this day on rejoicing in the deliverance that God has brought into your life. Tell others about that freedom and deliverance that you have been given. Write in the next section a proclamation that you are free.

SATURDAY EXPRESS OUR FREEDOM TO OTHERS:

Simply put, don't be silent. I am listening to the song by Steven Curtis Chapman called "live out loud." This is the message for today's study. You have been given new life and you should not be able to keep it inside you.

The line in the chorus to this song says the following... "Wake the neighbors, get the word out...kick up the music, climb a mountain and shout...this is life we been given, we should live it loud...so la la la la live out loud."

How true is this song? We should be living our freedom out loud for all to see. This was the reason for my writing this book.

As I spent the whole time of writing this book battling my own demons, I found that I had not told my story yet. I often would secretly speak of how God had helped me find freedom from obesity, but never openly. I would talk about how I wanted to go to a school and talk about struggling with my weight, but I still held back.

I am free! Why can I not declare this as truth?

John 8:36 New King James Version (NKJV)

36 Therefore if the Son makes you free, you shall be free indeed.

John 8:36 Amplified Bible (AMP)

36 So if the Son liberates you [makes you free men], then you are really and unquestionably free.

2 Corinthians 5:17 New King James Version (NKJV)

17 Therefore, if anyone is in Christ, he is a new creation; old things have passed away; behold, all things have become new.

2 Corinthians 5:17 Amplified Bible (AMP)

17 Therefore if any person is [ingrafted] in Christ (the Messiah) he is a new creation (a new creature altogether); the old [previous moral and spiritual condition] has passed away. Behold, the fresh and new has come!

Ephesians 1:3-14 New King James Version (NKJV)
Redemption in Christ

3 Blessed be the God and Father of our Lord Jesus Christ, who has blessed us with every spiritual blessing in the heavenly places in Christ,

4 just as He chose us in Him before the foundation of the world, that we should be holy and without blame before Him in love,

5 having predestined us to adoption as sons by Jesus Christ to Himself, according to the good pleasure of His will,

6 to the praise of the glory of His grace, by which He made us accepted in the Beloved.

7 In Him we have redemption through His blood, the forgiveness of sins, according to the riches of His grace

8 which He made to abound toward us in all wisdom and prudence,

9 having made known to us the mystery of His will, according to His good pleasure which He purposed in Himself,

10 that in the dispensation of the fullness of the times He might gather together in one all things in Christ, both[a]which are in heaven and which are on earth—in Him.

11 In Him also we have obtained an inheritance, being predestined according to the purpose of Him who works all things according to the counsel of His will,

12 that we who first trusted in Christ should be to the praise of His glory.

13 In Him you also *trusted,* after you heard the word of truth, the gospel of your salvation; in whom also, having believed, you were sealed with the Holy Spirit of promise,

14 who[b] is the guarantee of our inheritance until the redemption of the purchased possession, to the praise of His glory.

Ephesians 1:3-14 Amplified Bible (AMP)

3 May blessing (praise, laudation, and eulogy) be to the God and Father of our Lord Jesus Christ (the Messiah) Who has blessed us *in Christ* with every spiritual (given by the Holy Spirit) blessing in the heavenly realm!

4 Even as [in His love] He chose us [actually picked us out for Himself as His own] in Christ before the foundation of the world, that we should be holy (consecrated and set apart for Him) and blameless in His sight, *even* above reproach, before Him in love.

5 For He foreordained us (destined us, planned in love for us) to be adopted (revealed) as His own children through Jesus Christ, in accordance with the purpose of His will [[a]because it pleased Him and was His kind intent]—

6 [So that we might be] to the praise *and* the commendation of His glorious grace (favor and mercy), which He so freely bestowed on us in the Beloved.

7 In Him we have redemption (deliverance and salvation) through His blood, the remission (forgiveness) of our offenses (shortcomings and trespasses), in accordance with the riches *and* the generosity of His gracious favor,

8 Which He lavished upon us in every kind of wisdom and understanding (practical insight and prudence),

9 Making known to us the mystery (secret) of His will (of His plan, of His purpose). [And it is this:] In accordance with His good pleasure (His merciful intention) which He had previously purposed *and* set forth in [b]Him,

10 [He planned] for the maturity of the times and the climax of the ages to unify all things and head them up and consummate them in Christ, [both] things in heaven and things on the earth.

11 In Him we also were made [God's] heritage (portion) and we obtained an inheritance; for we had been foreordained (chosen and appointed beforehand) in accordance with His purpose, Who works out everything in agreement with the counsel and design of His [own] will,

12 So that we who first hoped in Christ [who first put our confidence in Him have been destined and appointed to] live for the praise of His glory!

13 In Him you also who have heard the Word of Truth, the glad tidings (Gospel) of your salvation, and have believed in and adhered to and relied on Him, were stamped with the seal of the long-promised Holy Spirit.

14 That [Spirit] is the guarantee of our inheritance [the firstfruits, the pledge and foretaste, the down payment on our heritage], in anticipation of its full redemption and our acquiring [complete] possession of it—to the praise of His glory.

I wrote all this scripture for the purpose of letting you see what, exactly, you have to share with others. So, many promises are filled throughout the scriptures. All of these belong to every believer.

There are so many other people that battle with obesity. So often these people carry other baggage. They struggle with depression and suicidal thoughts. They feel useless and worthless. Where are those believers that can simply tell them that God created them in His image and loves them with a boundless love?

Here is your walking paper, dear friend. Go forth and tell the world that God has set you free from the bondage of your demons. Tell them that you were created by the King of Glory and He loved you so much that He sent His own Son, Jesus, to die for you.

Tell them that they don't have to go through life feeling worthless. Tell them that God can set them free.

I leave you with this last passage from the Paul writing to the church at Ephesus. He tells them that it is the love of God that compels him to go through all the struggles that he has lived through. This is my heart for each person that struggles with obesity. This is my burden that I willingly carry with joy.

Ephesians 1:14-21 New King James Version (NKJV)

14 who[a] is the guarantee of our inheritance until the redemption of the purchased possession, to the praise of His glory.

Prayer for Spiritual Wisdom

15 Therefore I also, after I heard of your faith in the Lord Jesus and your love for all the saints,

16 do not cease to give thanks for you, making mention of you in my prayers:

17 that the God of our Lord Jesus Christ, the Father of glory, may give to you the spirit of wisdom and revelation in the knowledge of Him,

18 the eyes of your understanding[b] being enlightened; that you may know what is the hope of His calling, what are the riches of the glory of His inheritance in the saints,

19 and what is the exceeding greatness of His power toward us who believe, according to the working of His mighty power

20 which He worked in Christ when He raised Him from the dead and seated Him at His right hand in the heavenly places,

21 far above all principality and power and might and dominion, and every name that is named, not only in this age but also in that which is to come. Ephesians 1:14-21 Amplified Bible (AMP)

14 That [Spirit] is the guarantee of our inheritance [the firstfruits, the pledge and foretaste, the down payment on our heritage], in anticipation of its full redemption and our acquiring [complete] possession of it—to the praise of His glory.

15 For this reason, because I have heard of your faith in the Lord Jesus and your love toward all the saints (the people of God),

16 I do not cease to give thanks for you, making mention of you in my prayers.

17 [For I always pray to] the God of our Lord Jesus Christ, the Father of glory, that He may grant you a spirit of wisdom and revelation [of insight into mysteries and secrets] in the [deep and intimate] knowledge of Him,

18 By having the eyes of your heart flooded with light, so that you can know and understand the hope to which He has called you, and how rich is His glorious inheritance in the saints (His set-apart ones),

19 And [so that you can know and understand] what is the immeasurable and unlimited andsurpassing greatness of His power in and for us who believe, as demonstrated in the working of His mighty strength,

20 Which He exerted in Christ when He raised Him from the dead and seated Him at His [own] right hand in the heavenly [places],

21 Far above all rule and authority and power and dominion and every name that is named [above every title that can be conferred], not only in this age and in this world, but also in the age and the world which are to come.

This is the last study that I will leave you with. I hope that you will take this as an inspiration to find for yourselves a source for daily devotion. Do me one last favor and write your final thoughts from this week. Tell me if you understand the truth of RESTORE. Have you truly felt restored? Refreshed? Rebuilt?

RECIPE TIPS

I have gathered some recipes from friends and from my own ideas to help you with putting some imagination into your diet. Too often we pass up on a diet or give in to temptation simply out of diet boredom. Hopefully, these recipes will give you some ideas to put some zip into your meals.

So please use these as simply guidelines. I want to also acknowledge the resources that these recipes came from. At the end of this chapter I will list the recipe books and publishers that put all this vital information into my hands.

I will first go through the recipe books and lay out their ideas. These are individual dishes that are either based in chicken, beef, fish or vegetable ingredients.

These each have low fat, low cholesterol restrictions. These will also have some alternative ideas to keep your costs down to a minimum.

These first set of recipes come from the "Betty Crockers New low-fat, low cholesterol cookbook". This is published by Simon & Schuster Macmillan Company of New York, NY; copywrite 1996 by General Mills, INC.

Veal with Asparagus

4 servings (with about 1/2 cup vegetable mix each)
1 teaspoon vegetable oil
1 tablespoon finely chopped shallot
1 clove garlic, finely chopped
3/4 pound thin slices lean veal round steak or veal for scaloppini
1 cup sliced mushrooms (3 ounces)
1/3 cup dry white wine
2 teaspoons chopped fresh or 1/2 teaspoon dried thyme leaves
12 ounces asparagus spears, cut into 1-inch pieces

Heat oil in 10-inch nonstick skillet over medium-high heat. Cook shallot and garlic in oil, stirring frequently, until garlic is golden; reduce heat to medium. Add veal. Cook about 3 minutes, turning once, until light brown. Stir remaining ingredients. Heat until boiling; reduce heat. Cover and simmer about 12 minutes, stirring occasionally, until asparagus is crisp –tender

Caribbean Pork Tenderloin

4 servings (about 1 cup each)
The Plantain, a less-sweet cousin of the banana is a principal starch in the Caribbean. Tip: Partially freeze tenderloins to make it easier to slice them thinly.
2 lean pork tenderloins, about 1/2 lb each
1 teaspoon grated orange peel
1/2 cup orange juice
2 tablespoons chopped fresh cilantro
2 tablespoons lime juice
1/2 teaspoon cracked black pepper
2 cloves garlic, cut in half
1 teaspoon corn starch
1/4 teaspoon salt
1 teaspoon vegetable oil
1 large ripe plantain, cut into 1/4-inch slices

Trim fat from pork. Cut pork across grain into 1/8-inch slices. Mix orange juice, cilantro, lime juice, pepper and garlic in large glass or plastic bowl. Stir in pork. Cover and refrigerate 30 min.

Remove pork from marinade; drain, reserving marinade.

Stir cornstarch and salt into marinade; set aside. Heat oil in 10-inch nonstick skillet over medium-high heat. Cook pork in oil about 4 min. stirring frequently, until no longer pink. Stir in plantain. Cook 2 to 3 minutes, stirring frequently, until plantain is brown and slightly soft. Stir in marinade mixture.

Heat to boiling, stirring constantly. Boil and stir 1 minute.

Seasoned Pork Chops with Apples

4 servings (with 1/3 cup vegetable mixture each)
4 pork loin or rib chops, about 1/2 inch thick (about 1lb)
1/4 cup all-purpose flour
1 teaspoon chopped fresh or 1/2 teaspoon dried thyme leaves
1 teaspoon paprika
1/4 teaspoon pepper
1 1/2 cups fat-free chicken broth
2 cups sliced onions (about 1 large)
2 cups sliced cabbage
2 green apples, peeled and sliced
1/4 cup chopped fresh parsley

Trim fat from pork. Mix flour, thyme, paprika and pepper in plastic bag with zipper top. Add pork. Seal bag and shake until pork is well coated.

Heat oven to 350degree. Spray ovenproof Dutch oven with nonstick cooking spray. Heat Dutch oven over medium-high heat. Cook pork in Dutch oven until brown on both sides. Remove pork from Dutch oven.

Add broth to Dutch oven; scrape bottom with wooden spoon to loose any brown bits. Heat to boiling. Stir in onions and cabbage. Cook 5 minutes, stirring frequently. Top with pork and apples.

Cover and bake about 1 hour or until pork is tender. Sprinkle with parsley before serving.

Vegetable and Ham Jambalaya

6 servings (about 1 1/3 cups each)
A spunky rendition of the Louisiana specialty with only two grams of fat per serving.

3/4 cup fat-free chicken broth
1 medium onion, chopped (1/2 cup)
2 cloves garlic, finely chopped
1/2 cup diced green bell pepper
1/2 cup diced celery
2 green onions, chopped
4 cups cooked rice
1 cup frozen whole kernel corn or green peas
1 cup cubed lean fully cooked ham (about 2/3 lb)
1 tablespoon tomato paste
1 tablespoon Worcestershire sauce
1/2 to 1 teaspoon red pepper sauce
1 can (16 ounces) whole peeled tomatoes, undrained
1/3 cup chopped fresh parsley
1/2 teaspoon salt
1/2 teaspoon pepper

Heat broth to boiling in Dutch oven. Stir in onion, garlic, bell pepper, celery and green onions. Cook 5 to 8 minutes stirring frequently, until vegetables are tender.

Stir in remaining ingredients except parsley, salt and pepper, breaking up tomatoes. Heat to boiling, reduce heat to low. Cover and cook 30 minutes. Stir in parsley, salt and pepper. Serve with additional red pepper sauce if desired.

Ham with Cabbage and Apples

4 servings (with about 3/4 cup cabbage mixture each)
4 cups shredded cabbage
1 tablespoon packed brown sugar
1 tablespoon cider vinegar
1/8 teaspoon pepper
1 large green cooking apple, peeled, cored and cut into rings
1 medium onion, chopped (1/2 cup)
4 extra lean ham steaks (about 3 ounces each)

Spray 10-inch nonstick skillet with nonstick cooking spray. Cook all ingredients except ham in skillet over medium heat about 5 minutes, stirring frequently, until apple is crisp-tender.

Place ham on cabbage mixture; reduce heat to low. Cover and cook about 10 minutes or until ham is hot

Chicken Breasts with Sun-dried Tomato Sauce

4 servings (with about 1/3 cup sauce each)
Be sure to purchase the dried tomatoes that are not packed in oil.
1/4 cup coarsely chopped sun-dried tomatoes (not oil-packed)
1/2 cup fat-free chicken broth
4 boneless, skinless chicken breast halves (about 1 lb)
1/2 cup sliced mushrooms (1 1/2 ounces)
2 tablespoons chopped green onions
2 cloves garlic, finely chopped
2 tablespoons dry red wine or fat-free chicken broth
1 teaspoon vegetable oil
1/2 cup skim milk
2 teaspoons cornstarch
2 teaspoons chopped fresh or 1/2 teaspoon dried basil leaves
2 cups hot cooked fettuccine

Mix tomatoes and broth. Let stand 30 minutes.

Trim fat from chicken. Cook mushrooms, onions and garlic in wine in 10-inch nonstick skillet over medium heat about 3 minutes, stirring occasionally, until mushrooms are tender; remove mixture from skillet.

Add oil to skillet. Cook chicken in oil over medium heat until brown on both sides. Add tomato mixture. Heat to boiling; reduce heat. Cover and simmer about 10 minutes, stirring occasionally, until juice of chicken is no longer pink when centers of thickest pieces are cut. Remove chicken pieces from skillet; keep warm.

Mix milk, cornstarch and basil; stir into tomato mixture. Heat to boiling, stirring constantly. Boil and stir 1 minute. Stir in mushroom mixture; heat through. Serve over chicken and fettuccine.

Oriental Barbecued Chicken

4 Servings
Chicken thighs can be substituted for the breasts here, but they have about 9 milligrams more cholesterol per serving.
4 boneless, skinless chicken breast halves (about 1lb)
1/2 cup hoisin sauce
1 tablespoon sesame oil
1 tablespoon tomato paste
1/2 teaspoon ground ginger
2 cloves garlic, finely chopped

Set oven control to broil. Spray broiler rack with nonstick cooking spray.

Trim fat from chicken. Place chicken on rack in broiler pan. Mix remaining ingredients; brush on chicken.

Broil with tops about 4 inches from heat 7 to 8 minutes or until brown. Turn; brush with sauce. Broil 4 to 5 minutes longer or until juice of chicken is no longer pink when centers of thickest pieces are cut. Heat remaining sauce to boiling. Serve with chicken.

Curried Chicken and Nectarines

4 Servings (about 1 cup each)
4 boneless, skinless chicken breast halves (about 1lb)
2 tablespoons fat-free oil-and-vinegar dressing
1 teaspoon curry powder
1/4 cup raisins

1/4 cup sliced green onions (3 med)
1/4 teaspoon salt
1 med bell pepper, cut into 1/4-inch strips
2 small nectarines, cut into 1/4-inch slices
Hot cooked rice, it desired

Trim fat from chicken. Cut chicken crosswise into 1/2– inch strips. Mix dressing and curry powder in medium bowl. Add chicken; toss.

Heat 10-inch nonstick skillet over medium-high heat. Add chicken and remaining ingredients except nectarines and rice; stir-fry 4 to 6 minutes or until chicken is no longer pink in center. Carefully stir in nectarines; heat through. Serve with rice.

Thai Shrimp and Rice Noodle Nests

4 Servings (1/2 cup shrimp mixture and
1 cup noodle each)
Look for canned coconut milk marked "lite" when looking for reduced-fat coconut milk. Leftover milk can be frozen in small quantities for future uses.
1/4 cup finely chopped fresh basil leaves
1/4 cup Asian fish sauce or soy sauce
1/4 cup lime juice
2 tablespoons packed brown sugar
1 tablespoon cornstarch
1 lb uncooked peeled deveined med shrimp, cut into pieces
2/3 cup fat-free chicken both
6 cloves garlic, finely chopped
1 jalapeno chili, finely chopped
1 cup julienned broccoli stems or flowerets
2/3 cup shredded carrot (1 med)
2/3 cup finely chopped red or green bell pepper
1/4 cup chopped fresh cilantro
3 tablespoons reduced-fat coconut milk
4 cups hot cooked rice noodles or linguine

Mix basil, fish sauce, lime juice, brown sugar and cornstarch in shallow glass or plastic dish. Stir in shrimp. Cover and refrigerate 20 minutes.

Heat broth to boiling in nonstick wok or 10-inch skillet. Add garlic, chili and broccoli; stir-fry 5 to 8 minutes or until broccoli is crisp-tender. Add carrot and bell pepper; stir-fry 3 minutes. Add shrimp and marinade; stir-fry 3 to 5 minutes or until shrimp are pink and sauce thickens slightly. Stir in cilantro and coconut milk; remove from heat.

Coil 1 cup noodles in center of each plate. Top with 1/2 cup shrimp mixture.

The following list of recipes come from the book "Betty Crockers New Eat and Lose Weight." This book is published by Simon and Schuster Macmillan Company in New York, NY, copyright @1996 by General Mills, Inc.

I would suggest that you pick this up to find some additional ideas for recipes.

Orange and Ginger Glazed Chicken

4 Servings
Spreadable fruits contain no added reined sugar, but instead rely on the sugar within various fruits for sweetness.
4 boneless, skinless chicken breast halves (about 1lb)
1/3 cup orange marmalade speadable fruit
1 teaspoon finely chopped gingerroot or 1/2 teaspoon ground ginger
1 teaspoon Worcestershire sauce

Spray 10-inch skillet with nonstick cooking spray; heat over medium-high heat. Cook chicken in skillet about 5 minutes or until bottoms are brown; turn chicken. Stir in remaining ingredients; reduce heat to low.

Cover and simmer 10 to 15 minutes, stirring sauce occasionally, until sauce is thickened and juice of chicken is no longer pink, when centers of thickest pieces are cut. Cut chicken into thin slices. Spoon sauce over chicken.

Garlic Chicken Kiev

6 Servings
3 tablespoons reduced-calorie spread, softened
1 tablespoon chopped fresh chives or parsley
1/8 teaspoon garlic chicken breast halves (1 1/2 lb)
2 cup cornflakes, crushed (about 1cup)
2 tablespoons chopped fresh parsley
1/2 teaspoon paprika
1/4 cup low-fat buttermilk or skim milk

Mix spread, chives and garlic powder; shape into rectangle, 3X2 inches. Cover and freeze about 30 minutes or until firm. Trim fat from chicken. Flatten each chicken breast half to 1/4-inch thickness between waxed paper or plastic wrap.

Heat oven to 425 degree. Spray square pan, 9X9X2 inches, with nonstick cooking spray. Cut chives mixture crosswise into 6 pieces. Place 1 piece on center of each chicken breast half. Fold long sides of chicken over chives mixture; fold up ends and secure with toothpick.

Mix cornflakes, parsley and paprika. Dip chicken into buttermilk, then lightly and evenly coat with cornflake mixture. Place chicken, seam sides down, in pan. Bake uncovered about 35 minutes or until chicken is no longer pink in center.

Ginger Chicken with Curried Couscous

4 Servings
1 tablespoon reduced-sodium soy sauce

1 tablespoon honey
1 tablespoon grated gingerroot
4 skinless boneless chicken breast halves (1lb)
2 1/4 cups ready-to-serve fat-free reduced-sodium chicken broth
1 1/4 cups uncooked couscous
4 medium green onions, sliced (1/4 cup)
3/4 teaspoon curry powder

Mix soy sauce, honey and ginger root in shallow nonmetal dish or heavy-duty resealable plastic bag. Add chicken; turn to coat. Cover dish or seal bag and let stand 20 min at room temperature.

Heat broth to boiling in 10-inch nonstick skillet. Stir in couscous, onions and curry powder; remove from heat. Cover and let stand 8 to 10 minutes or until broth is absorbed.

Meanwhile, set oven control to boil. Place chicken on rack in broiler pan. Broil with tops 1 inch from heat 5 minutes; turn. Broil about 3 minutes longer or until juice is no longer pink when centers of thickest pieces are cut. Serve over couscous.

Chicken Nicoise

4 Servings
A small amount of olives and a bouquet of herbs lend exotic flavor to this traditional dish from Nice, France. Usually made with tuna fish, out chicken version puts a new spin on an old classic.
1 1/4 cups dry white wine or ready-to-serve fat-free reduced-sodium chicken broth
4 skinless boneless chicken thighs or breasts (1lb)
3 cloves garlic, fined chopped
1/2 cup frozen pearl onions
1 tablespoon Italian seasoning

2 medium bell peppers, sliced
6 chopped pitted Kalamata olives (2 onions)
2 cups hot cooked rice

Heat 1/4 cup of the wine to boiling in 10-inch nonstick skillet. Cook chicken in wine, turning once, until brown. Remove chicken from skillet, keep warm.

Add garlic, onions, Italian seasoning, bell peppers, olives and remaining 1 cup wine to skillet. Heat to boiling; boil 5 minutes. Add chicken; reduce heat to medium. Cook 10 to 15 minutes or until juice of chicken is no longer pink when centers of thickest pieces are cut. Serve over rice.

Orange Roughy with Red Peppers

4 Servings
1 lb orange roughy, walleye or sole fillets
1 teaspoon olive or vegetable oil
1 small onion, cut into thin slices
2 medium red bell peppers, cut into julienne strips
1 tablespoon chopped fresh or 1 teaspoon dried thyme leaves
1/2 teaspoon salt
1/4 teaspoon pepper

If fish fillets are large, cut into 4 serving pieces. Heat oil in 10-inch nonstick skillet over medium heat. Layer onion and bell peppers in skillet . Sprinkle with half of the thyme and pepper. Layer fish on bell peppers. Sprinkle with remaining thyme, salt and pepper. Reduce heat to medium. 5 to 10 minutes longer or until fish flakes easily with fork.

Louisiana Seafood Creole

4 Servings

Packaged frozen vegetable and canned tomatoes make this flavorful supper dish a snap.

1/2 cup dry white wine or ready-to-serve fat-free reduced-sodium chicken broth
3 cups frozen green beans, red peppers, and carrots (from 16-ounce package)
4 large cloves garlic, finely chopped (1 tablespoon)
1/4 to 1/2 teaspoon ground red pepper (cayenne)
1/2 lb cod, halibut or red snapper fillets, cubed
1 can (16 ounces) stewed tomatoes, undrained
1 lb uncooked, peeled, deveined small shrimp, thawed if frozen
Hot cooked rice, if desired

Heat 1/4 cup of the wine to boiling in 4-quart Dutch oven or saucepan.

Stir in vegetable mixture and garlic. Cook about 10 minutes, stirring frequently,

until liquid has evaporated. Stir in remaining wine, the red pepper, fish and

tomatoes. Heat to boiling; reduce heat to medium. Cover and cook 20 minutes.

Stir in shrimp. Cook about 5 to 7 minutes or until shrimp are pink and firm.

Serve over rice.

Beef Medallions with Pear-Cranberry Chutney

4 Servings
Bright and tangy, this easy fruit chutney sets off the hearty beet. Serve leftover chutney cold on a turkey sandwich, or try it with chicken as well.
1 large red onion, thinly sliced
2 cloves garlic, finely chopped
2 tablespoons dry red wine or grape juice
2 firm ripe pears, peeled and diced
1/2 cup fresh or frozen cranberries
2 tablespoons packed brown sugar
1/2 teaspoon pumpkin pie spice
4 beef tenderloin steaks, about 1 inch thick (1 lb)

Spray 2-quart saucepan with nonstick cooking spray; heat over medium-

high heat. Cook onion, garlic and wine in saucepan about 5 minutes, stirring

frequently, until onion is tender but not brown. Stir in remaining ingredients except beef. Simmer uncovered, stirring frequently, until cranberries burst. Place chutney in small bowl; set aside.

Meanwhile, spray 10-inch nonstick skillet with nonstick cooking spray; heat over medium-high heat. Cook beef in skillet about 8 minutes, for medium doneness, turning once. Serve with chutney.

Pork Medallions: Trim fat from pork. Cut pork crosswise into 12 slices; flatten slightly. Follow directions above for Pear-Cranberry Chutney. Meanwhile, spray 10-inch skillet with nonstick cooking spray; heat over medium-high heat. Cook pork in skillet about 8 to 10 minutes turning once, or until pork is slightly pink in center. Serve with chutney.

I am including some ideas of my own into this recipe guide. I hope it will give you some enjoyment.

Low-Fat High Protein Smoothie

2 servings
This is a great quick snack idea. It is best to have this prior to a workout time. The high protein of the egg whites will help with energy and muscle development
2 cups low-fat or skim milk
4 cups crushed ice
1 cup of fresh fruit (apples, bananas, cherries, etc)
1 1/2 tablespoons of honey or apple sauce (to sweeten)
1 egg white

Blend milk, ice, egg white until mixed thoroughly. Add fruit and honey to taste. Blend until completely smooth. Serve in chilled glass.

Big Mouth Burgers

4 servings
The following is a burger idea that I have used for many years. I have adapted this recipe to be more health conscious.

Understand that the name came from the fact that my hands are of above average size. Therefore the name was attached saying that you had to have a big mouth to eat one. So I will try and reflect this in measurements.

1 lb of lean ground beef, turkey, or steak
1/4 teaspoon garlic powder
1/4 teaspoon salt
1/4 teaspoon pepper
1/2 white onion chopped fine
1/2 green bell pepper, diced small
1 tablespoon Worcestershire sauce
1 can sliced mushrooms
1 cup mixed shredded cheese to taste
1 thinly sliced fresh tomato
1 thinly sliced fresh white onion

Place garlic powder, salt, pepper, chopped onion, diced pepper all in large bowl. Mix together and add meat. Combine dry ingredients thoroughly into the meat then add Worcestershire sauce, mushrooms, and cheese.

Pre-heat 10-inch skillet at medium-high heat. Spray nonstick fat-free cooking spray onto skillet.

Remove enough meat to cover your palm. Keep patty approximately an inch thick. Place patty onto skillet and cook until lightly brown or to taste.

Brown wheat hamburger buns in toaster oven. Cover one side of bun with fat-free mayonnaise, relish, ketchup, a slice of onion, a slice of tomato and fresh lettuce. Drain patty and place on the bun.

Serve with a bowl of fresh fruit and a glass of water.

There are many resources available for those who are seeking to create a collection of low-fat, low-sodium, high-protein recipes. All it takes is doing some research and asking friends.

Feel free to experiment with the recipes that you have used in the past. Substitute your usual ingredients with low-fat or low-sodium ingredients.

You will notice that I used apple sauce in exchange for sugar. This is a great way to add some zip to oatmeal or to cold cereal. It adds sweet without adding the processed sugar.

Another substitute would be adding yogurt instead of sugar. This also helps add protein. However, be aware of the fat content and do not use per-flavored yogurt.

FINAL THOUGHTS

This book has been a growth for myself and hopefully for you, my reader. I have been honest and open to you as I have struggled with my own demons. I hope that you will step into a new freedom and life after putting this book back on the shelf.

I want to let you know that I would enjoy hearing from each of you as you move closer to that place of complete freedom. Send me pictures and letters to tell me how this book has helped you.

I would also like to hear from anyone that wants to add to this work with their own personal life story. Tell me how God has brought you from bondage to freedom. I will include in this last passage a collection of photos that I hope will give you encouragement.

I am amazed at how God has brought me through so much in working on this project. It truly had become an obsession. The most amazing part of this whole thing is that I grew up hating exercise and now I find that I feel guilty because I haven't been in the gym in a while.

I hope that you, dear reader, will reach the same point in your life. I hope that you will find your life so radically changed that you can become another "fitness fanatic".

The most important part that I hope you bring from reading through this book is that I pray you have been healed, emotionally.

Too many of us have carried around baggage that holds us in bondage and I hope that you have found freedom. Do me a favor and take the time to tell someone near you what has happened in your life? Make this a message to help others experience true freedom from the past.

I leave you with a group of scriptures that express to you my heart. Because during this whole time of writing this book I have battled through a great war in my own life. After eighteen years, I have lost my marriage. Much of the reason for this is due to my own issues. But I have found myself falling back into old habits that I have told you to lay aside.

I apologize for my hypocrisy. But I am being honest with you and telling you that I haven't achieved success completely yet. But God is faithful and has carried me through the darkest point in my life. I want you to know that God will carry you when you cannot take another step.

Take this last chapter and read through these passages. I hope that you will find comfort in the hard times from these passages. Just step into the reality and you will find freedom.

This is an excerpt from my book, "Mountain Moving Faith" and it tells the truth of what I have learned through all of my struggle over the past year. I hope it helps close off this book the right way.

Remember that God can work through the most impossible situation in your life. Even when the doctor tells you to just accept your size and don't try to change. When he tells you to be satisfied with just 10 or 20 pounds. Read through this passage and I feel you will be encouraged.

In our surrender we must now let God have freedom to do whatever He chooses to do. He must have full control of our lives, our finances, our children, our work, etc. As we do this we must begin to praise God for what He is about to do. This means no matter what it may be, and even before we see the results of His move.

The Word of God is filled with people of God facing impossible situations and standing in faith. From the Old Testament through the New Testament, we are told time after time how God proved Himself true.

Daniel saw the mouths of the lions shut. Abraham was promised a son and received one in his old age. Samson fought an army single handed and defeated them. David faced Goliath with three stones and took his head.

The best story that presents this truth though is the story of the three Hebrew children as they stood before the king.

Now let me lay out the setting of our three Heroes of Faith. The king Nebuchadnezzar had sent out orders that the people of the land had to bow and worship him at the sound of the trumpet. The consequence of not bowing would be death.

However, there were three Hebrews that refused to bow, despite the potential consequences. Well, the king was royally upset. He ordered that they were to be arrested and brought before him.

Daniel 3:13-18 New King James Version (NKJV)

13 Then Nebuchadnezzar, in rage and fury, gave the command to bring Shadrach, Meshach, and Abednego. So they brought these men before the king.

14 Nebuchadnezzar spoke, saying to them, "*Is it true*, Shadrach, Meshach, and Abednego, *that* you do not serve my gods or worship the gold image which I have set up?

15 Now if you are ready at the time you hear the sound of the horn, flute, harp, lyre, *and* psaltery, in symphony with all kinds of music, and you fall down and worship the image which I have made, *good!* But if you do not worship, you shall be cast immediately into the midst of a burning fiery furnace. And who *is* the god who will deliver you from my hands?"

16 Shadrach, Meshach, and Abednego answered and said to the king, "O Nebuchadnezzar, we have no need to answer you in this matter.

17 If that *is the case,* our God whom we serve is able to deliver us from the burning fiery furnace, and He will deliver *us* from your hand, O king.

18 But if not, let it be known to you, O king, that we do not serve your gods, nor will we worship the gold image which you have set up."

Daniel 3:13-18 Amplified Bible (AMP)

13 Then Nebuchadnezzar in rage and fury commanded to bring Shadrach, Meshach, and Abednego; and these men were brought before the king.

14 [Then] Nebuchadnezzar said to them, Is it true, O Shadrach, Meshach, and Abednego, that you do not serve my gods or worship the golden image which I have set up?

15 Now if you are ready when you hear the sound of the horn, pipe, lyre, trigon, harp, dulcimer or bagpipe, and every kind of music to fall down and worship the image which I have made, very good. But if you do not worship, you shall be cast at once into the midst of a burning fiery furnace, and who is that god who can deliver you out of my hands?

16 Shadrach, Meshach, and Abednego answered the king, O Nebuchadnezzar, it is not necessary for us to answer you on this point.

17 If our God Whom we serve is able to deliver us from the burning fiery furnace, He will deliver us out of your hand, O king.

18 But if not, let it be known to you, O king, that we will not serve your gods or worship the golden image which you have set up!

I want you to see these key phrases in this passage. This is crucial to allowing God to work in your impossible situation. Look at the power of their faith. They accepted that it was not what they wanted. They were completely submitted to the will of God.

Now, understand that they told the king that it wasn't a decision that they took lightly. They had spent time praying about this. They knew the potential result was death. Yet, this did not sway their decision.

What consequence are you willing to face to follow the will of God in this situation? Are you willing to loose your home, your friends, your family, your life?

Daniel 3:19-25 New King James Version (NKJV)
Saved in Fiery Trial

19 Then Nebuchadnezzar was full of fury, and the expression on his face changed toward Shadrach, Meshach, and Abednego. He spoke and commanded that they heat the furnace seven times more than it was usually heated.

20 And he commanded certain mighty men of valor who *were* in his army to bind Shadrach, Meshach, and Abednego, *and* cast *them* into the burning fiery furnace.

21 Then these men were bound in their coats, their trousers, their turbans, and their *other* garments, and were cast into the midst of the burning fiery furnace.

22 Therefore, because the king's command was urgent, and the furnace exceedingly hot, the flame of the fire killed those men who took up Shadrach, Meshach, and Abednego.

23 And these three men, Shadrach, Meshach, and Abednego, fell down bound into the midst of the burning fiery furnace.

24 Then King Nebuchadnezzar was astonished; and he rose in haste *and* spoke, saying to his counselors, "Did we not cast three men bound into the midst of the fire?" They answered and said to the king, "True, O king."

25 "Look!" he answered, "I see four men loose, walking in the midst of the fire; and they are not hurt, and the form of the fourth is like the Son of God."[a] Daniel 3:19-25 Amplified Bible (AMP)

19 Then Nebuchadnezzar was full of fury and his facial expression was changed [to antagonism] against Shadrach, Meshach, and Abednego. Therefore he commanded that the furnace should be heated seven times hotter than it was usually heated.

20 And he commanded the strongest men in his army to bind Shadrach, Meshach, and Abednego and to cast them into the burning fiery furnace.

21 Then these [three] men were bound in their cloaks, their tunics *or* undergarments, their turbans, and their other clothing, and they were cast into the midst of the burning fiery furnace.

22 Therefore because the king's commandment was urgent and the furnace exceedingly hot, the flame *and* sparks from the fire killed those men who handled Shadrach, Meshach, and Abednego.

23 And these three men, Shadrach, Meshach, and Abednego, fell down bound into the burning fiery furnace.

24 Then Nebuchadnezzar the king [saw and] was astounded, and he jumped up and said to his counselors, Did we not cast three men bound into the midst of the fire? They answered, True, O king.

25 He answered, Behold, I see four men loose, walking in the midst of the fire, and they are not hurt! And the form of the fourth is like a son of the gods!

The faith of these three men carried them up to and through the ultimate sacrifice. Yet they did not waver. But now, after they have overcome the king, the result is to walk through the fire with the Son of God.

But lets get this whole thing down to our individual lives. How can we see God walk with us midst our fiery furnace? We must first realize that we are not longer looking at our situation through earthly eyes. We need to look through the eyes of faith.

This means that we need to tap into the authority that we have in the Name of Jesus Christ. David spoke of the proving of the armor. We have proven the armor of God and found it faithful. Read through 'role call of faith' found in the book of Hebrews and you can see how He has proven faithful.

1 Samuel 17:34-37 New King James Version (NKJV)

34 But David said to Saul, "Your servant used to keep his father's sheep, and when a lion or a bear came and took a lamb out of the flock,

35 I went out after it and struck it, and delivered *the lamb from* its mouth; and when it arose against me, I caught *it* by its beard, and struck and killed it.

36 Your servant has killed both lion and bear; and this uncircumcised Philistine will be like one of them, seeing he has defied the armies of the living God."

37 Moreover David said, "The LORD, who delivered me from the paw of the lion and from the paw of the bear, He will deliver me from the hand of this Philistine." And Saul said to David, "Go, and the LORD be with you!"

1 Samuel 17:34-37 Amplified Bible (AMP)

34 And David said to Saul, Your servant kept his father's sheep. And when there came a lion or again a bear and took a lamb out of the flock,

35 I went out after it and smote it and delivered the lamb out of its mouth; and when it arose against me, I caught it by its beard and smote it and killed it.

36 Your servant killed both the lion and the bear; and this uncircumcised Philistine shall be like one of them, for he has defied the armies of the living God!

37 David said, The Lord Who delivered me out of the paw of the lion and out of the paw of the bear, He will deliver me out of the hand of this Philistine. And Saul said to David, Go, and the Lord be with you!

David was functioning in faith based upon what he had seen God do in his life, time and again. Sadly, Saul should have been able to move in the same faith. The Hebrew tradition of that time was to pass on the history of their families from one generation to another. Yet the army of Israel sat on the ridge in fear.

Saul had long since forgotten the power of the God of his forefathers. He had long since forgotten the great acts of people like Abraham, Moses, Isaac, and others.

But, sadly there are many of us who have done the very same thing. We've forgotten the God of our forefathers. We've place God into a box of tradition, ritual and religion. We have declared that this is as far as He can move and no further.

We need to remove those walls and recognize that we serve the same God that spoke the worlds into existence. ***We serve the God who raised Lazarus, closed the lions mouth, delivered a nation, killed a giant, rebuilt a nation, birthed out Savior, split the temple veil, rose from the dead, and gave us salvation, healing, deliverance, restoration, and a promised returning Glorious King.***

Hebrews 12:1-2 New King James Version (NKJV)
The Race of Faith
12 Therefore we also, since we are surrounded by so great a cloud of witnesses, let us lay aside every weight, and the sin which so easily ensnares us, and let us run with endurance the race that is set before us,

2 looking unto Jesus, the author and finisher of our faith, who for the joy that was set before Him endured the cross, despising the shame, and has sat down at the right hand of the throne of God.

Hebrews 12:1-2 Amplified Bible (AMP)
12 Therefore then, since we are surrounded by so great a cloud of witnesses [who have borne testimony to the Truth], let us strip off and throw aside every encumbrance (unnecessary weight) and that sin which so readily (deftly and cleverly) clings to and entangles us, and let us run with patient endurance and steady and active persistence the appointed course of the race that is set before us,

2 Looking away [from all that will distract] to Jesus, Who is the Leader and the Source of our faith [giving the first incentive for our belief] and is also its Finisher [bringing it to maturity and perfection]. He, for the joy [of obtaining the prize] that was set before Him, endured the cross, despising and ignoring the shame, and is now seated at the right hand of the throne of God.

So I bid to you a farewell and good fighting.

Know that you do serve a great God and He did not create you by accident. You have purpose in life that no man or thing or demon or situation or circumstance can change that purpose. Every event, every person, every crisis in your life has come to you by the hand of a mighty and loving God.

I will let you ponder this one thing from the book "Purpose Driven Life." In the book the author tells us how we were created for a purpose. But have you ever considered that God hand picked your parents simply for the purpose to create you. They possessed the exact DNA that He chose to make you. They held the genetic material needed to shape you the way that God wanted.

That puts our obesity into a whole new light. That tells us that we may have impaired the creation that God had in plan but it still is there and He can still work out His will in our life. Go now and fulfill the purpose that God has for you. Pick up that book, "Purpose Driven Life" and read through it as you work the program. You will find God opening your eyes to a new vision of your life.

Thank you for reading my book and I hope and believe that God will bless you. Randy.